AVERY

SOY PROTEIN

WHAT YOU NEED TO KNOW

MARY CAROLE McMANN, MPH, RD, LD

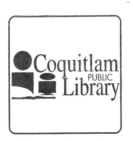
AVERY

a member of PENGUIN PUTNAM INC.   New York

Most Avery books are available at special quantity discounts for bulk purchase for sales promotions, premiums, fund-raising, and educational needs. Special books or book excerpts also can be created to fit specific needs. For details, write Putnam Special Markets, 375 Hudson Street, New York, NY 10014.

Avery
a member of
Penguin Putnam Inc.
375 Hudson Street
New York, NY 10014
www.penguinputnam.com

ISBN: 0-89529-988-7

Printed in the United States of America

10 9 8 7 6 5 4 3 2 1

This book is printed on acid-free paper. ∞

Series Cover Designer: Doug Brooks
Cover Image Courtesy of PhotoDisc

CONTENTS

INTRODUCTION

Prevention is a key word in health care today. It has taken a long time for both the healthcare system and the general public to accept the importance of *preventing* disease, instead of just attempting to repair the damage once disease has occurred. Part of working toward prevention involves identifying the underlying causes of certain diseases. Epidemiologists investigate disease trends in various areas of the world and study the differences in the rates of certain chronic illnesses. Epidemiological studies have found that Asian countries have lower rates of several chronic diseases that are major killers in the West. Many of these research projects have led epidemiologists to look at differences in diet, in hopes that preventive factors can be identified.

Of course, there are many differences between Western eating and the traditional Asian diet. Asian peoples tend to eat less fat and to consume more fruits and vegetables than individuals who eat higher-fat Western cuisines. But researchers felt that these factors still didn't fully explain the differences in rates of chronic disease between East and West. So they turned to a staple of many Asian cuisines that is almost completely lacking in most Western diets—the mighty soybean. Soybeans and various soyfoods made from them are important components of Asian eating. The soybean is a major protein source in Eastern food patterns, which typically contain little or no animal sources of protein—meat, fish, poultry, eggs, and dairy products.

Until recently, the only people in the United States who seemed interested in soyfoods and soy protein were individuals following a vegetarian diet. Vegetarians typically had to search out a fairly limited number of soyfoods available only in health food and other specialty food stores. But, in recent years the story of soy and soy protein has taken an exciting new turn. Information about the health benefits of soy protein has been showing up in mainstream magazines and other publications. As a result, a growing number of traditional soyfoods and newer foods containing soy-protein ingredients have become widely available.

There are a number of important reasons why many Americans have begun to take a closer look at soy protein:

- The growing global population makes it increasingly important to consider protein sources that are lower on the food chain, that is, that require less of our limited natural resources to produce.

- A new and improved method for evaluating protein quality shows that certain forms of soy protein are equal in quality to protein in milk, egg white, and meat.

- Health authorities recommend adopting a diet based primarily on plant foods, including legumes such as soybeans, fruits, vegetables, grains, and nuts. For example, the U.S. Department of Agriculture's (USDA) Food Guide Pyramid, the Dietary Guidelines for Americans, and nutrition recommendations of the American Cancer Society and the American Heart Association all emphasize eating more complex-carbohydrate foods from plant sources, including soy.

- A great deal of research on the health benefits of phytochemicals—substances naturally occurring in plant foods—has focused on the isoflavones found almost exclusively in soy. Research suggests that soy isoflavones may help prevent several chronic diseases that plague Western nations.

Because the information on soy and soy protein is growing so rapidly, it can be difficult to tell fact from fiction. The purpose of this book is to provide the most up-to-date, accurate information on what we know about the health benefits of soy protein. Chapter 1 explains what makes soy such a healthy food and covers soy protein, soy isoflavones, and other components of soy. Chapters 2 through 5 each discuss a particular disease or health issue—cardiovascular disease, cancer, osteoporosis, and menopause-related problems, respectively—and explore the way that soy protein with naturally occurring isoflavones may help prevent or treat the conditions. Chapter 6 tells you exactly what you need to know to make soy protein a part of your daily diet. It describes various sources of soy protein and makes some suggestions about amounts you might want to include in your diet. Finally, a glossary of key health and nutrition terms and a list of helpful references are also included to provide you with further information.

So take a step toward better health now and in the future. Find out all you have to gain by adding soy protein with naturally occurring isoflavones to your diet.

1

WHAT MAKES SOY SO SPECIAL?

There are a number of important reasons why soy is so special. First, soy represents the only plant source of protein that is as high in quality as animal protein. Second, research indicates that soy may have exciting health benefits in helping prevent a number of chronic diseases. Third, soybeans are a very versatile food that can be consumed in a growing number of tasty forms. The majority of Americans are just now becoming aware of what Asian peoples have known for years: soy is both good and good for you!

THE FASCINATING HISTORY OF SOY

Soy may be relatively new to you, but it's one of the oldest foods in recorded history. It is believed that the soybean was first derived from a legume native to central China. (Legumes are plants with seed-bearing pods that are higher in protein than other plants.) Soybeans were cultivated as a crop in the eleventh century B.C., and by 300 B.C. they had become a major food crop in northern China. Soybeans have been used in China for more than 5,000 years, not only as food, but as components of medicine. The Chinese considered soybeans to be one of their most important crops, identifying soy as one of the five sacred grains necessary for life.

The growth of soybeans slowly spread throughout all of China and into Japan, Korea, and Southeast Asia. The soybean appeared in Japan in the seventh century A.D., where it became a staple of Japanese cuisine—a role soyfoods still play today. No one actually knows how soybeans made their way to Europe around the seventeenth century. Perhaps they were used as ballast (something used to add weight) in trading vessels coming from China, keeping the ships steadier in the water. As Western missionaries and traders returned from Asia, they may have brought tofu (soybean curd) back to their native countries.

Soybeans and other soyfoods most likely came to the United States with Chinese immigrants in the early 1800s. However, soyfoods remained primarily a part of Eastern cuisine until around the turn of the twentieth century, when early advocates of vegetarianism began to develop and promote soy-based alternatives to milk and meat. By the early part of the twentieth century, scientists were already investigating possible roles of soy in the treatment of diabetes and anemia, as well as in the feeding of infants with milk allergies.

United States farmers began growing soybeans in 1829, and by 1917 they were planting about 50,000 acres in soybeans. By 1996, soybean production in the United States had grown to more than 64 million acres. Although soybeans have become an important food crop in this country, half of the soybeans grown in the United States are exported, and much of the rest is used for animal feed. Yet there is a steady growth in the consumption of soyfoods in the United States.

Between 1980 and 1996, for example, the production of tofu grew by 128 percent, and soymilk production increased by almost 5,800 percent! During this same period, the total pounds of soy ingredients produced for human consumption—soy flour, textured soy flour, soy protein concentrates, and isolated soy protein—increased by 146 percent. What is exciting all of this new interest in soyfoods? One major factor is the increasing number of reports suggesting that soy may have beneficial effects on several chronic diseases and conditions.

A quick look at current health statistics shows that people in Japan and other Asian countries have lower rates of the chronic diseases that are major killers in Western nations, namely heart disease and cancer. Women in the East also have lower rates of osteoporosis—a disease in which bones become weak and brittle. Furthermore, Asian women experience fewer symptoms when they reach menopause. Since these health advantages tend to disappear when Asians move to the West, researchers have studied lifestyle factors that often change during the Westernization process. One of these is diet.

The traditional Asian diet is lower in fat and higher in fiber than most Western cuisines. Even when these dietary habits are taken into account, however, they don't appear to explain all of the differences in the incidence of chronic diseases between East and West. So researchers began to look at another essential difference between Eastern and Western eating patterns— soyfoods—and began conducting in-depth studies on the components that make soy so special.

SOY PROTEIN

Soy protein is a mainstay of Asian diets, which typically are either vegetarian or contain what, by American standards, are considered to be very small amounts of animal-protein foods. In traditional Asian cuisines, meat, fish, poultry, eggs, and dairy products are usually side dishes, rather than entrees. Therefore, the protein in soy has a long history of playing a primary roll in fulfilling protein's most basic functions in the human body. In fact, soy provides up to 60 percent of the total dietary protein in some Southeastern Asian countries.

Protein makes up about 38 to 42 percent of the soybean. The actual percent protein that is present depends on a number of factors, including the variety of soybean and its growing conditions. Similarly, soyfoods and soy ingredients provide differing amounts of protein. Soy margarine, soy sauce, and soy oil contain no protein. But many soy products are rich in this essential nutrient. Table 1.1 gives several examples of soy products and lists their protein content. You can get soy protein from soyfoods such as tofu or soymilk, or in a soy ingredient that you add to recipes or that is incorporated in a commercial soy-based food product. The soy ingredients

Table 1.1. Soy Protein in Common Soyfoods and Soy Ingredients

Soyfood/Soy Ingredient	Serving Size	Protein (grams/serving)
Soy protein isolates*	1 ounce	26.1
Soybean seeds, dry roasted (dry roasted soynuts)	$\frac{1}{4}$ cup	17.0
Soy protein concentrate	1 ounce	16.5
Tofu, soft	1 cup, $\frac{1}{2}$″ cubes	16.2
Mature soybeans, cooked	$\frac{1}{2}$ cup	14.3
Soy flour, defatted	$\frac{1}{4}$ cup, stirred	11.8
Green soybeans, cooked	$\frac{1}{2}$ cup	11.1
Tofu, firm	$\frac{1}{2}$ cup	10.1
Soymilk	1 cup	6.7

* Value is for *Supro* brand soy protein isolates from Protein Technologies International, St. Louis, MO. All other values are from the United States Department of Agriculture (USDA) Nutrient Database for Standard Reference.

typically used in commercial soyfood products are soy protein concentrates and soy protein isolates.

Soy protein concentrates are made from defatted soy flakes. They are about 70 percent protein and retain most of the dietary fiber in the soybean. Soy protein concentrates are usually processed using an alcohol extraction method (see page 9 for more information).

At 92 percent protein, isolated soy protein (ISP), sometimes called soy protein isolates, is the most refined source of soy protein available. ISP is made by removing protein from defatted soy flakes, typically using a water extraction method. Water extraction tends not to remove isoflavones—beneficial plant chemicals (discussed later)—to the extent resulting from alcohol extraction. Furthermore, some ISP is processed using special techniques to keep isoflavone loss at a minimum, so that you can reap the benefits of both soy protein and its isoflavones.

The Importance of Protein

Why is there so much emphasis on the protein in soy? Well, protein is a vital part of all living tissues. Its primary functions are to build new tissue during periods of growth and healing, and to repair and maintain the tissues of the body. Protein is made up of building blocks called *amino acids.* There are twenty amino acids needed by the human body. The body can synthesize more than half of the twenty, but there are nine amino acids that it is not capable of producing. These amino acids, called *essential amino acids,* must be supplied in your food.

Food proteins are often classified as complete or incomplete. Complete food proteins contain all of the essential amino acids in the amounts necessary to carry out protein's functions in the body. Incomplete proteins are those food proteins that lack sufficient amounts of one or more of the essential amino acids. In the past, it was thought—and taught—that all animal proteins (except gelatin) were complete and that all plant proteins were incomplete. Vegetarians were advised to combine complementary protein sources within a meal. This means they were instructed to consume two or more incomplete protein foods that together provide all of the essential amino acids. A familiar example is the popular combination of red beans and rice. Combining incomplete protein foods within one meal is no longer emphasized. Research has shown that the total amino acids consumed throughout the day are what's important. Furthermore, soy protein is now recognized as a complete protein.

The Quality of Soy Protein

For years, nutritionists and other health professionals maintained that soy protein was superior to other plant proteins, but inferior to the proteins found in meat, fish, poultry, dairy products, and eggs. The first part of this belief is true; the second part is not.

Protein quality is evaluated by comparing the amino acid profile of a food protein with a standard amino acid profile, which reflects the amino acid needs of a particular reference group. Until recently, the Protein Efficiency Ratio (PER) was the preferred method for establishing protein quality, and the PER rated soy protein as providing insufficient amounts of several essential amino acids. The standard amino acid profile used in PER, however, was based on the amino acid requirements of young rats, not of growing humans. For example, the PER reflects the need for a higher level of methionine, an amino acid that rats require in greater amounts to support the growth of body hair. Because soy protein didn't provide enough methionine to support hair growth in rats, the PER rated it as inferior to animal protein sources.

Then Protein Digestibility-Corrected Amino Acid Scoring (PDCAAS) was developed. PDCAAS is based on several factors: a food protein's profile of essential amino acids; the digestibility of the protein; and the protein's ability to supply essential amino acids in the amounts needed to meet the requirements of growing human beings. In 1993, the Food and Drug Administration (FDA), following the lead of the Food and Agricultural Organization/World Health Organization (FAO/WHO), adopted PDCAAS as the standard for calculating the percent Daily Value of protein used on food labels for adults and for children over the age of one year. As is shown in Table 1.2 on page 8, the more accurate PDCAAS methodology shows certain forms of soy protein to be equivalent in quality to casein (milk protein), egg white, and beef protein.

The highest possible PDCAAS is 1.0. This is because once the body's need for protein to build and repair tissues has been met, excess amino acids aren't used as protein; they are either burned as fuel or stored.

SOY ISOFLAVONES

Without a doubt, the most exciting area of nutrition research today is that of phytochemicals. The term *phytochemical,* which simply means "plant chemical," refers to thousands of different compounds naturally found in plant foods. Phytochemicals are not vitamins or minerals. However,

Table 1.2. Protein Digestibility-Corrected Amino Acid Scoring for Selected Food Proteins

Protein Source*	PDCAAS
Soy protein isolate†	1.00
Casein (milk protein)	1.00
Egg white	1.00
Beef protein	0.92
Pea flour	0.69
Kidney beans (canned)	0.68
Pinto beans (canned)	0.63
Whole wheat	0.40

*Protein Quality Evaluation, Report of the Joint FAO/WHO Expert Consultation. Rome: FAO Food and Nutrition, Paper No. 51, 1989.

†Values for *Supro* brand soy protein isolate provided by Protein Technologies International, as determined through actual analysis.

research continues to discover new potential health benefits associated with consuming them.

Because of the explosion of knowledge in this area of nutrition, research investigating potential health benefits of soy has increasingly been focused on its phytoestrogens. *Phytoestrogens* are a group of phytochemicals that perform some estrogen-like activities in the body. For example, women consuming larger amounts of the phytoestrogens in soy tend to have less osteoporosis and fewer or less severe menopausal symptoms. One type of phytoestrogen found in foods is a family of compounds called *isoflavones.*

Isoflavones are one type of phytochemical found in soy, and soy is a major source of these phytoestrogens in the human diet. The major isoflavones in soy are genistein, daidzein, and glycitein. Genistein, in particular, has come under extensive study because of its various potentially healthy activities.

Soyfoods differ in their isoflavone contents for several reasons. Each soybean crop may contain a different amount of isoflavones, depending on the variety of soybean being raised, the growing conditions, the soil, and the season in which the soybean crop is harvested.

Isoflavones occur naturally with soy protein. However, it is important to note that some extraction methods used to manufacture soy protein concentrates and soy protein isolates can affect the isoflavone content. An alcohol-based extraction method, such as is typically used in the processing of soy protein concentrates, removes alcohol-soluble compounds naturally found in soy—including isoflavones. Extensive water extraction can also remove isoflavones, but processing methods have been developed that can keep the naturally occurring isoflavones intact. Be sure to select products that contain a reliable brand of soy protein ingredients.

It is important to keep in mind that soy protein contains many other biologically active components in addition to isoflavones. As our knowledge increases, it is possible researchers will discover that components other than isoflavones, but present along with them in soy protein, are responsible for some or all of the effects being observed in studies.

SOY FIBER

For years now, you have been hearing about the importance of fiber in the diet. You probably remember the extensive publicity about oat bran's role in lowering cholesterol. The component that was found to be responsible for this effect is *soluble fiber.* The other major type of fiber—*insoluble fiber*—is also important to health because it plays a role in normal elimination of solid waste from the body. Soy fiber is about 30 percent soluble fiber, the remaining fiber being insoluble. Some research suggests that soy fiber may have a modest cholesterol-lowering effect in people with elevated blood-cholesterol levels.

OTHER COMPONENTS OF SOY

There are several other components of soy that are being investigated for their potential contribution to soy's exciting health benefits. Among these are specific amino acids in soy protein, soy globulins, phytic acid, saponins, and a type of protease inhibitor. These areas of study are briefly discussed below. More research is needed before we can arrive at any definitive conclusions on how these components affect our health.

Amino Acids

Some research has investigated whether particular amino acids in soy protein might have an effect on cholesterol levels. One example is the amino acid lysine. Studies have shown that lysine increases cholesterol levels in animals. When the amino acids present in soy protein are compared with those in milk protein, the soy protein has a lower level of lysine. This is discussed in more detail in Chapter 2 (page 15). Although studies in animals have shown that feeding the exact amino acids found in soy protein results in lower cholesterol levels, the cholesterol reduction is greater when these same amino acids are fed as intact soy protein. This difference in response suggests that there are other biologically active components in soy protein that most likely play a role in cholesterol lowering.

Soy Globulins

Most of the protein in soy is in the form of globulins. The two major soy globulins in soybeans—11S and 7S—have been studied to see if they might have a role in soy's ability to lower cholesterol. Research in animals indicates that 7S may help lower cholesterol.

Phytic Acid

Soy contains phytic acid, which binds to minerals, decreasing the absorption of zinc, calcium, iron, and magnesium in the body. People eating a diet with a high level of zinc in relation to copper may have an increased tendency for elevated blood-cholesterol levels. One theory is that phytic acid's ability to decrease zinc absorption may allow more copper to be absorbed, thereby helping to lower cholesterol levels. Some animal studies suggest that phytic acid may play a role in lowering cholesterol, but by a different mechanism. Currently, researchers are not positive how the phytic acid in soy influences cholesterol.

Saponins

Saponins are compounds found in association with plant protein. Some animal studies suggest that the addition of saponins to a diet containing animal protein may lower cholesterol levels. However, research doesn't currently support the theory that saponins can account for soy's cholesterol-lowering ability.

Protease Inhibitor

Soy also contains a particular type of protease inhibitor, called the Bowman-Birk inhibitor. Protease is an enzyme that has a role in breaking down protein during digestion. Studies in the laboratory and in animals suggest that the Bowman-Birk inhibitor found in soy may partially or totally affect the transformation of normal cells to cancerous ones (see page 20).

A WORD ABOUT RESEARCH

The information contained in this book is gathered from various types of studies. Often, preliminary information comes from epidemiology—the study of the causes, distribution, and control of disease in populations. However, population studies can't prove cause and effect; in other words, they can't prove that the factor, such as diet, either causes the disease, has no effect on it, or helps prevent it. Epidemiological observations provide the hints that lead to more specific types of research.

Laboratory, or *in vitro,* research is conducted in an artificial environment, such as a test tube. *In vivo* studies, on the other hand, are conducted in living organisms, including animals and humans. Whenever possible, the studies cited in this book will be *in vivo* studies in humans. Any other *in vivo* studies are identified as being in animals.

CONCLUSION

Soybeans and other traditional soyfoods have had a very long history of safe and beneficial consumption by millions of people. The protein in soy is the only plant protein equal in quality to animal protein sources. In addition, soy and soy protein contain other naturally occurring substances with potential health benefits, especially soy isoflavones. The following chapters will examine what is currently known about soy and specific health conditions.

2

CARDIOVASCULAR DISEASE

A considerable amount of the research investigating soy protein has focused on cardiovascular disease (CVD). CVD, which includes heart attack, stroke, and high blood pressure, is the number one killer of American men and women, accounting for more than 41 percent of all deaths. It is estimated that half of these deaths are the result of coronary heart disease, primarily heart attack. CVD touches the life of every American, either directly or indirectly—through personal loss and/or the considerable financial cost of these diseases to society. It is estimated that in 1999, CVD will cost the United States $286.5 billion in direct health costs and lost productivity.

Although CVD represents a major cause of death in many nations, statistics are not uniform in all areas of the world. For example, a look at the most recent worldwide statistics show that the death rate (number of deaths per 100,000 population) from CVD in the United States is 413 for men and 201 for women, but in Japan, the death rate is 201 for men and 99 for women. There are a number of factors that may contribute to such a significant difference. Diet is certainly one of them. In comparing Eastern and Western diets, researchers have turned to the study of soy. Before we look at the research being done to investigate soy and heart health, it is important to understand the basics of heart disease, particularly the type of damage to arteries that is a major cause of most heart attacks.

ATHEROSCLEROSIS—THE HIDDEN MENACE

An elementary understanding of atherosclerosis is important to any discussion of heart disease because it is the underlying process in the vast majority of heart attacks. Basically, *atherosclerosis* is characterized by changes in the wall of an artery—the type of blood vessel that carries blood away from the heart and delivers it throughout the body. A normal artery is flexible. As the heart contracts, it pumps blood into the artery, which is able to expand in response to the increased internal pressure from the rush of blood. The artery then contracts and becomes smaller between heartbeats, when the heart is relaxed. An atherosclerotic artery is unable to adequately carry out these expansions and contractions.

The most widely accepted theory is that atherosclerosis occurs when an artery is injured. For example, high blood pressure can lead to artery damage. The body then starts the repair process, but something goes awry. A fatty substance, called cholesterol (see below), and other materials in blood are deposited on the surface and in the interior of the artery wall, making it thicker and more rigid. This process is often described as "hardening" of the artery. Plaque—material deposited in and on the artery wall—usually builds up gradually, taking years, even decades, to get to the point where a noticeable problem occurs in the cardiovascular system.

As plaque accumulates, the opening inside the artery becomes narrower, decreasing the amount of blood that is able to reach the cells beyond. If the artery becomes totally blocked, the flow of blood is cut off and the tissues "fed" by that artery are damaged and may even die. In many cases, the complete blocking of an atherosclerotic artery is the result of a blood clot, which forms in or on the surface of the plaque or is carried by the bloodstream from somewhere else in the body. The blood clot acts like a cork in a narrow-necked bottle.

When an artery inside the heart itself becomes clogged, the result is a heart attack. The seriousness of a heart attack depends on the size of the area affected by the blockage, as well as the specific region of the heart that is damaged. When an artery is blocked in the neck or the head, a stroke occurs. Atherosclerosis is the underlying cause of about 70 to 80 percent of all strokes.

Heart attacks and strokes are usually the end results of a series of events. The level of cholesterol in the blood helps determine the growth of plaque in the artery (see below for more information). Other factors contributing to blocked arteries include the decreased ability of an atherosclerotic artery to expand in response to the pressure from blood flowing through it and the person's increased tendency to form blood clots.

THE CHOLESTEROL CONNECTION

Cholesterol is a fatty, waxy substance that has several important functions in the human body. For example, it is vital to the structure of every cell in the body. It also is a building block that your body uses to make several types of hormones. Many people are only aware of cholesterol's negative side—it is the substance that makes up a large proportion of artery-clogging plaque.

Cholesterol is a type of fat, while blood is primarily water. And just like oil and water, the two don't mix. In order for cholesterol to travel around in your bloodstream, it is combined with protein to make a particle called a *lipoprotein*. How the cholesterol in your blood influences your health greatly depends on the type of lipoprotein in which it is contained. The two most familiar lipoproteins are low-density-lipoprotein (LDL) and high-density-lipoprotein (HDL). A high level of LDL-cholesterol in the blood is considered a major risk factor for heart disease because it is associated with increased plaque growth and a greater risk of heart attack. HDL-cholesterol is another story. It not only doesn't increase your chances of having a heart attack, it actually decreases your risk. When the level of HDL-cholesterol is too low, your risk of heart attack goes up.

SOY PROTEIN AND CHOLESTEROL LOWERING

There are two primary ways that soy protein with naturally occurring isoflavones may protect against the damage done by LDL-cholesterol. Soy isoflavones not only help reduce LDL-cholesterol levels in the blood, they also act as antioxidants.

Direct Cholesterol-Lowering Effect

Studies in animals and in humans have investigated the cholesterol-lowering ability of soy protein. In the summer of 1995, Dr. James W. Anderson and his associates published a landmark meta-analysis of the effects of soy protein on lipoprotein levels in the blood. (A meta-analysis uses statistical methods to combine the results of a number of smaller studies.) The meta-analysis, which appeared in *The New England Journal of Medicine,* analyzed the combined data from thirty-eight clinical studies, which together included 730 research volunteers. It showed that replacing animal protein with soy protein resulted in a 9.3 percent decrease in total cholesterol, a 12.9 percent decrease in LDL-cholesterol, and a 10.5 percent decrease in triglyceride, which is another blood fat associated with CVD. All of these decreases were statistically significant. The individuals who originally had the highest blood-cholesterol levels experienced the greatest degree of cholesterol lowering.

The meta-analysis had two major effects. First, it raised public awareness of soy protein's potential health benefits in CVD. Second, it spurred what has become a steadily increasing interest in investigating soy and soy protein among members of the research and medical communities. The next logical question was: what component or components in soy lowers cholesterol?

Research has shown that some particular amino acids tend to raise blood cholesterol levels, and others help to lower them. As was briefly mentioned in Chapter 1, the amino acid lysine increases cholesterol levels in animals. In contrast, the amino acid arginine decreases cholesterol. It has been suggested that the lower level of lysine and the higher level of arginine found in soy protein, when compared with casein (milk protein), help explain why soy has a greater cholesterol-lowering effect. It is important to note that animals fed soy protein experienced a greater degree of cholesterol lowering than those fed a purified mixture of the same amino acids found in soy. This difference suggests that there is something in soy protein over and above the specific amino acids present that causes soy protein to lower cholesterol.

As was also mentioned in Chapter 1, there has been some research indicating that soy globulins (storage proteins) lower blood-cholesterol levels. However, a growing number of studies have provided convincing evidence of the importance of soy protein containing naturally occurring isoflavones. Remember, there is still a possibility that some other biologically active component or components present in soy protein may be responsible for some of the effects attributed to isoflavones.

Researcher Mary Anthony and her associates investigated the effects in monkeys of two soy-protein diets—one with naturally occurring isoflavones and the other with the isoflavones mostly removed. They compared these two groups with monkeys fed a diet containing casein, the principal animal protein in dairy products. Of the three groups, the monkeys receiving the soy protein with naturally occurring isoflavones had significantly lower blood-cholesterol levels and had the highest HDL-cholesterol levels. (Remember, a high level of HDL-cholesterol is desirable.) This study and other studies in monkeys by the same researchers suggest that the isoflavones in soy may be critical in the cholesterol-lowering effects of soy protein.

Researchers have also looked at the effects in humans of soy protein containing different levels of naturally occurring isoflavones. Crouse and colleagues conducted a study to clarify whether the naturally occurring isoflavones in soy are critical to its cholesterol-lowering effect in humans. Study subjects, who had moderately elevated LDL-cholesterol levels, were divided into five groups. All subjects received 25 grams of protein per day.

One group consumed animal protein (casein), a second group consumed soy protein with almost all of the isoflavones removed, and three groups consumed soy protein containing different levels of naturally occurring isoflavones. The subjects who consumed casein or the soy protein without isoflavones had no significant change in their levels of total or LDL-cholesterol. The three groups consuming soy protein with isoflavones decreased their blood-cholesterol levels. The greatest degree of cholesterol lowering was achieved in the group consuming soy protein with the highest level of naturally occurring isoflavones. The cholesterol lowering was greater in those individuals with the highest initial blood-cholesterol values. The study demonstrated that soy protein with isoflavones lowers blood cholesterol in humans and that the effect is dose-dependent—that is, it increases as the isoflavone content goes up.

The effects of extracted isoflavones have recently been investigated. When menopausal and perimenopausal (during three to five years before menopause) women consumed a purified soybean extract that contained only isoflavones, they failed to lower their blood-cholesterol levels. All of these studies help show that soy protein with naturally occurring isoflavones lowers blood-cholesterol levels, that soy protein without isoflavones does not lower blood cholesterol, and that isoflavones without soy protein also do not lower blood cholesterol.

You don't need to consume a lot of soy protein to get the benefits. The people with high cholesterol levels who were included in the Anderson meta-analysis (see page 14) consumed an average of 47 grams of soy protein per day. However, another often quoted study by Bakhit and associates showed that men with elevated cholesterol levels had a significant decrease in blood cholesterol when they consumed as little as 25 grams of soy protein per day. So, it really isn't that difficult to consume the amount of soy protein necessary to start gaining benefits.

Antioxidant Effect

The cholesterol story doesn't end there. It is now widely accepted that not all LDL-cholesterol acts the same way in the body. LDL-cholesterol that has been damaged by a chemical reaction called *oxidation* is the major contributor to the atherosclerotic process. This is one reason there has been such a growth in interest in substances that act as *antioxidants,* that is, substances that can help protect molecules (such as LDL-cholesterol molecules) from being oxidized.

Genistein and daidzein, two of the main isoflavones found in soy, are thought to act as antioxidants. *In vitro* studies have shown that both of these isoflavones may reduce the oxidation of LDL-cholesterol.

On a side note, there is growing interest in the possible role of antioxidants in minimizing the adverse effects of exercise. Research has shown that oxidation reactions during exercise can contribute to your being tired and sore, and may increase your chances of being injured. In one study by Rossi, DiSilvestro, and colleagues, young men consumed either a whey-based product or a soy beverage containing genistein twice a day for three weeks. The study showed that the soy beverage improved antioxidant activity both before and after exercise; the whey beverage had no effect. The soy group had an increase in total antioxidant status in the blood before exercise. General antioxidant actions were also evident in the soy group after exercise, and members of this group had lower multiple indicators of oxidant stress. For example, the group consuming soy had a smaller increase in creatine kinase, an enzyme that indicates muscle injury, suggesting that soy protein may decrease exercise-induced fatigue, soreness, and injury. Further studies are anticipated to confirm these findings.

MORE POTENTIAL HEART HEALTH BENEFITS OF SOY PROTEIN

There are a number of other factors in addition to cholesterol that affect the growth of atherosclerotic plaque and the blocking of arteries in the heart. New research suggests that soy protein with naturally occurring isoflavones may also have a positive effect on some of these factors.

Effect on Atherosclerosis

As part of the study in monkeys described on page 15, Anthony and her colleagues also measured the plaque in the coronary arteries of some of the monkeys. The arteries of the monkeys receiving soy protein with naturally occurring isoflavones had 90 percent less atherosclerosis compared with the casein group, and 50 percent less compared with the group receiving soy protein with most of the isoflavones removed. The researchers could not determine whether the partial benefit seen in the monkeys consuming soy protein essentially without isoflavones was due to traces of isoflavones remaining in the soy protein or to some other component of soy protein.

Effect on Artery Dilation

Normal arteries are able to dilate (enlarge) in response to a neurotransmitter called acetylcholine. (A neurotransmitter is a chemical agent released by an "excited" nerve cell. It crosses the very tiny area—synapse—

between nerve cells and stimulates the next cell in the nerve.) However, acetylcholine has an opposite effect on atherosclerotic arteries; it causes them to constrict, or become smaller. Honoré and associates conducted studies in monkeys to investigate the effect of soy protein with and without naturally occurring isoflavones on the ability of an atherosclerotic artery to dilate. The researchers found that soy protein with naturally occurring isoflavones improved dilation in response to acetylcholine in arteries of female monkeys fed a diet that caused atherosclerosis. The arteries of the female monkeys not receiving isoflavones and both groups of male monkeys continued to constrict in response to acetylcholine.

Effect on Smooth Muscle Cells

The rapid reproduction of smooth muscle cells in artery walls is essential to the growth of atherosclerotic plaque. Phytoestrogens, such as isoflavones, have been shown to inhibit this rapid reproduction. Some studies suggest that genistein may act in this way, inhibiting several of the steps in the initiation and formation of atherosclerotic plaque.

Effect on Blood Clotting

Another area of interest in heart research is the formation of blood clots, which stimulate the growth of atherosclerotic plaque. *In vitro* studies have shown that genistein potentially interferes with many aspects of the blood-clotting system that are believed to promote plaque growth. Further studies are needed to see if genistein also exhibits these activities in animals and in humans.

Effect on Restenosis

An important problem associated with heart disease is restenosis—the reappearance of narrowing in an atherosclerotic artery after medical efforts have been made to open the artery. Restenosis often occurs following a process called percutaneous transluminal coronary angioplasty (PTCA), which involves inserting a catheter with a tiny balloon in its tip into the atherosclerotic artery and positioning it at the site of a partial blockage. The balloon is then inflated and withdrawn, to compress the plaque and enlarge the inner diameter of the artery.

Studies in animals showed that estradiol, a very potent form of estrogen produced in the body, inhibited the thickening of the artery lining in response to a balloon injury. This led researchers to investigate the possible effects of phytoestrogens, such as soy isoflavones, on the artery. Honoré and associates conducted a study in which female monkeys were fed diets designed to cause atherosclerosis. One diet contained soy protein with naturally occurring isoflavones, while the second soy-protein diet had most of the isoflavones removed. The atherosclerotic arteries of the monkeys were then injured by a balloon. The researchers found that restenosis was inhibited in the animals that consumed the diet containing soy protein with isoflavones.

CONCLUSION

It is important for us to make lifestyle changes that can help reduce the risk of developing cardiovascular disease. One area of continuing interest is diet. Research has shown that soy protein with naturally occurring isoflavones reduces levels of LDL-cholesterol in the blood. Since oxidized LDL-cholesterol actually does the damage to your arteries, it is important that the isoflavones naturally occurring in soy protein may also act as antioxidants—preventing, reducing, or regulating this oxidative damage. And, research is investigating other ways in which soy protein with naturally occurring isoflavones may contribute to heart health. In light of all these possible benefits from consuming soy, a growing number of health-conscious people are choosing to make soy products a regular part of their daily diets.

3

CANCER

A lthough cancer is the second largest killer in the United States, it is the disease most dreaded by Americans. Health authorities have begun to focus more of their attention on prevention by identifying lifestyle factors that increase or decrease the risk of developing cancer. Diet has been identified as a critical factor in many types of cancer. Researchers are now investigating the potential role of soy and soy protein in preventing specific cancers. First, it is important to understand how this disease starts and spreads.

CANCER BASICS

Cancer is a general term referring to a large group of diseases that all have one thing in common—abnormal cells growing and multiplying in an uncontrolled manner, often spreading throughout the body. Cancer isn't like an infectious disease, in which one exposure to bacteria or a virus may result in illness. It first has an *initiation phase* during which a normal cell in the body is damaged, making it abnormal. In this phase, a *carcinogen*—a cancer-causing agent—changes the very nature of the cell by altering its genetic material, or DNA. Common carcinogens include things that exist both inside and outside the body. Smoking, chemicals, extended exposure to sunlight, radiation, and viruses are examples of external carcinogens. Internal carcinogens include hormones, immune conditions, abnormal cells that are inherited, and the oxidation process that occurs in your body every day.

Your immune system neutralizes or destroys untold numbers of potentially cancerous cells every day. Therefore, how well your immune system is functioning may have an impact on your likelihood of developing cancer. In addition, cancer cells produce special proteins, called stress proteins, that help them survive normal cell destruction (see page 23). It is only in the second phase, called *promotion,* that a damaged, or "initiated," cell actually becomes cancerous.

Normal cells in your body multiply and develop into cells with specialized functions, and they do so in an orderly and controlled fashion. Cancer occurs when there is damage to the genes that control normal cell division. In the promotion phase of cancer development, a promotional agent causes cancerous cells to divide and multiply until they crowd out neighboring normal cells, taking the nutrients they need. Cancerous cells can grow into a solid mass, called a *tumor,* and they may spread throughout the body in a process called *metastasis.*

Epidemiologists have noted that some types of cancer are less common in Asian countries, such as Japan and China, than in Western nations, including the United States. Among these are hormone-dependent cancers such as breast and prostate cancers. Table 3.1 lists the death rates from breast and prostate cancers in selected Eastern and Western countries.

Table 3.1. Death Rates Per 100,000 Population for Selected Cancers

Country	Breast Cancer	Prostate Cancer
Western Nations		
United States	21.1	17.3
United Kingdom	26.5	17.1
Germany	22.1	16.9
Eastern Nations		
Japan	6.8	5.0
China	4.2	Not available

Originally, it was thought that the low fat content of the Asian diet explained the differences in cancer rates between East and West. Although the higher fat content in the American diet may be associated with an increased risk of certain cancers, the hypothesis that fat actually causes cancer has not been supported by clinical trials. Next, researchers considered the other side of the coin—that something or, more likely, several things in the Asian diet might help protect against cancer. This has led to a number of studies investigating foods that are characteristic of the Asian diet, including soy. When the National Institutes of Health sponsored a symposium in late 1994 to report on the disease-prevention qualities of plant foods, at least two-thirds of the presentations mentioned genistein, the primary isoflavone in soy and soy protein.

SOY PROTEIN AND CANCER

There are a growing number of studies suggesting that soy and/or naturally occurring soy isoflavones have anticancer activity. Of course, it is still possible that one or more other biologically active components present with isoflavones in soy protein may be responsible for some of these results. In 1994, for example, a review of twenty-six studies evaluated the effect of soy or soy isoflavones on eight cancer sites in animals. A majority of the studies (seventeen of twenty-six, or 65 percent) showed that soy may have a protective effect. Although researchers have not identified any one mechanism to explain soy's potential anticancer activity, much of the focus has been on soy isoflavones.

The following sections discuss several processes and substances naturally occurring in the body that may play a role in the development of cancer, along with how soy may affect them. The processes include oxidation, malfunctions in the immune system, and angiogenesis. The substances include stress proteins, hormones, and tyrosine kinases.

Oxidation

The chemical process of oxidation is one of the ways that cells in your body can be damaged and become cancerous. Oxidation occurs when oxygen reacts with another substance to produce free radicals—very reactive particles capable of damaging DNA to produce potentially cancerous cells. Some studies have suggested that the *antioxidant* properties of genistein—that is, its ability to reduce the cell damage done by oxidation—might have an anticancer effect.

Immune System Function

As was mentioned previously, your immune system has the job of destroying or neutralizing potentially cancerous cells in your body. Researchers have looked at possible effects of soy protein isoflavones on the immune system. One recent study showed that high doses of daidzein, the second most plentiful isoflavone in soy protein, enhanced the functioning of the immune system in mice. Zhang and the other researchers who conducted the study suggested that this enhancement of immune function might help explain the contribution of soyfoods to cancer prevention.

Angiogenesis in Cancer

A promising new area of cancer research has to do with a process called angiogenesis, which consists of the development of tiny new blood vessels.

Whenever the body undergoes growth, it must provide new blood vessels to supply the oxygen and nutrients needed to nourish the developing area. Under normal circumstances, angiogenesis rarely occurs in adults; the exceptions are during wound healing and as part of the menstrual cycle.

Since cancer cells require a blood supply to support their uncontrolled multiplication, increased angiogenesis is a basic requirement of tumor growth. Research suggests that substances that inhibit angiogenesis could prevent the nourishment of a tumor, essentially acting as a tourniquet and limiting the ability of the tumor to grow beyond the size of a pea. Although antiangiogenic substances can't prevent cancer, they may be able to stop a tumor from growing very large. In *in vitro* studies, genistein has been found to be a potent inhibitor of angiogenesis.

Stress Proteins

Most cells in the body have a limited life span built into their genetic code. However, when the cells are threatened by stress conditions, such as viral infections, inflammations, and the onset of cancer, they can cause the synthesis of special proteins called stress proteins. These proteins protect the cells, including cancerous cells, against normal programmed cell death, which allows the cancerous cells to survive longer than healthy cells. Researchers Zhou and Lee found evidence that genistein may inhibit this stress response in both cancerous and precancerous cells *in vitro*. In fact, they described genistein as "an anticancer phytoestrogen from soy."

Hormones

The potential effects of soy-protein isoflavones on hormone-dependent cancers, such as breast and prostate cancers, have been investigated. The activities of both natural and synthetic estrogens depend upon their binding to estrogen receptors in different body tissues. Isoflavones are considered estrogen agonists, which means that they can bind to estrogen receptors and act in much the same way as estrogens. However, there are some important differences.

Isoflavones bind weakly to estrogen receptors, when compared with more potent estrogens. In addition, once an isoflavone is bound to an estrogen receptor, it has much less estrogenic activity than other estrogens—both natural and synthetic. It is estimated that genistein has only about .001 the estrogen activity of *estradiol*, a highly potent, naturally occurring form of estrogen. These less potent effects are desirable, since breast cancer is associated with the degree of estrogen activity at the receptor.

Isoflavones can also act as *antiestrogens,* or *estrogen antagonists.* (An antagonist neutralizes or interferes with the action of another agent, such as estrogen.) High levels of synthetic estrogens in the body appear to be counteracted by isoflavones, whether obtained from the diet or administered separately. The ability of isoflavones to reduce the effect of estrogens suggests that they may potentially be useful in the prevention of hormone-dependent tumors.

Another way isoflavones in soy protein affect hormones has to do with sex hormone-binding globulin (SHBG). As the name suggests, SHBG is a protein that binds to sex hormones, making them unavailable for hormonal activities in the body. Research has shown that isoflavones may stimulate synthesis in the liver. This increase in SHBG not only lowers the percentage of free estradiol in the body, but also reduces its biological activity.

Tyrosine Kinases

Tyrosine kinases are enzymes that play an essential role in the series of cell changes that lead to the development of cancer. Agents with the ability to inhibit the activity of tyrosine kinases have long been recognized as having anticancer properties. One mechanism for genistein's potential anticancer activity may be associated with its role as an inhibitor of tyrosine kinases.

CANCER SITES OF SPECIAL INTEREST

Researchers who are studying the possible role of soy protein with naturally occurring isoflavones in cancer prevention have focused primarily on tumors known to be affected by hormones and diet. Most of these studies have investigated cancers of the breast, prostate, uterus, or stomach.

Breast Cancer

Among American women, breast cancer is the most common cancer and the second leading cause of cancer death. (Lung cancer is the number-one killer.) An estimated 175,000 new cases of invasive breast cancer are expected to occur in women in 1999, and about 1,300 new cases will be diagnosed in men. (Invasive cancers are those that have begun to spread to other parts of the organ or to other sites in the body.) Breast cancer is expected to kill an estimated 43,300 women and 400 men in 1999.

Epidemiological evidence suggests that the length of time breast tissue is exposed to estrogen may be associated with breast cancer risk. The longer the menstrual cycle, the less time breast tissue is exposed to estrogen. This has led researchers to look at the effect of eating soyfoods on the length of the menstrual cycle in healthy women. One study by Lu and associates showed that consuming soyfoods containing phytoestrogens increased the length of the menstrual cycle and decreased blood levels of certain hormones, including a type of estradiol. These effects are known to influence both the multiplication of breast cancer cells and breast cancer risk. In this study, the longer menstrual cycle and lowered level of estradiol persisted even after the soyfood diet was discontinued.

Furthermore, in a number of studies, genistein has been shown to inhibit cell growth in both hormone-dependent and hormone-independent breast cancer cells *in vitro*. The mechanism by which genistein inhibited the growth of breast cancer cells isn't known. More research is needed in order to better understand this effect of genistein.

Lamartiniere and associates conducted studies in which genistein was given to rats either directly after their birth (during the neonatal period) or before puberty. Two groups of rats used as control animals were given dimethylsulfoxide (DMSO). All of the rats were later exposed to a chemical agent known to cause breast cancer. Both groups of rats that received genistein had fewer tumors and experienced a longer period of time before the tumors appeared—an increased latency period.

The important thing to keep in mind is that soy isoflavones are chemically similar to naturally occurring and synthetic forms of estrogen. They are able to compete with more potent forms of estrogen at estrogen receptors, but have much less estrogenic activity. Research suggests that soy isoflavones are able to mimic some of estrogen's functions, such as helping prevent bone loss, but may not stimulate the unfavorable responses in breast tissue that may increase the risk of cancer.

Prostate Cancer

Prostate cancer is the most common cancer among American men, accounting for an estimated 179,300 new cases in 1999. Cancer of the prostate is the second leading cause of cancer death in men. (Again, lung cancer is first.) It will cause the deaths of an estimated 37,000 men in 1999.

Some interesting information from China has thrown a new light on how soy protein may contribute to the lower death rate from prostate cancer in Asian men, when compared with that of Western men. Autopsies have revealed that Chinese men have about *half* the number of tiny (microscopic) prostate tumors as are found in men in Western countries, including the United States. However, the incidences of clinical prostate cancer and death from prostate cancer are *twenty* times less in China than in the United

States! These data suggest that one of the reasons the rates of developing active prostate cancer are so much lower in China is that these men have a higher incidence of very small inactive, or dormant, tumors. There is no direct evidence to explain these vast differences in the incidence of prostate cancer and in rates of prostate cancer death between Chinese and Western men.

Researchers speculate that the isoflavone genistein may inhibit both the promotional phase of cancer development and angiogenesis (see page 22). This has caused some leading epidemiologists who specialize in nutrition and eating habits to suggest that there may be an association between soyfood consumption in China and the higher incidence of tiny, "clinically silent" prostate tumors in Chinese men. This hypothesis will bear further investigation.

Furthermore, researchers conducting *in vitro* studies have found that genistein decreases the growth of both hormone-dependent and hormone-independent prostate cancer cell lines. A study in rats with prostate cancer conducted by Schleicher and associates showed that genistein injections inhibited tumor growth and delayed the spread of tumors. It remains to be seen if this positive effect can be demonstrated in human studies.

Whenever substances with potential hormonal activity, such as isoflavones, are added to the diet, there is always concern about the possibility of increasing hormone levels and promoting the growth of hormone-dependent cancers. For this reason, as part of a study in male rhesus monkeys, Anthony and associates looked at the effect of feeding soy protein either with or without soy isoflavones on testosterone levels and on the weight of the prostate and testicles. They found that the diet containing naturally occurring isoflavones had no effect on testosterone level. The two groups of monkeys had no substantial differences between the weight of their prostates or testicles. An increase in the weight of an organ is a possible indicator of cancer. The researchers concluded that their data support the hypothesis that soy estrogens are specific for certain tissues—that is, they don't have the same effects in all the tissues in the body. In part, this is thought to be due to the fact that isoflavones can act both as estrogen agonists and as estrogen antagonists.

In an interesting side note, genistein also appears to inhibit the growth of noncancerous prostate tissue, the cause of an enlarged prostate. This disorder, called benign prostatic hypertrophy or benign prostatic hyperplasia (BPH), occurs in approximately 20 percent of men aged forty-one to fifty years, and increases to over 80 percent in men older than eighty years.

Uterine Cancer

It is estimated that in 1999, there will be about 37,400 new cases of uterine cancer, primarily cancer of the endometrium (the membrane lining the inside of the uterine wall). Uterine cancer is expected to cause about 6,400 deaths in this same year. Death rates from this type of cancer tend to range from a little to a lot lower in Asian countries, when compared with the United States and European countries. According to data from the American Cancer Society, the death rates from uterine cancer (other than cervical cancer) are 2.5 in the United States, 2.2 in the United Kingdom, 3.0 in Germany, 2.1 in Japan, and 0.7 in China.

Researchers are investigating a possible role for soy in helping prevent uterine cancer. Goodman and his associates conducted a study in which they identified an association between soy consumption and a decreased risk of endometrial cancer, especially in women who did not use estrogen replacement therapy (ERT).

ERT has been associated with an increased risk of endometrial cancer. This has raised the question of whether or not phytoestrogens, including soy isoflavones, might have a similar effect. In an *in vivo* study, female rhesus monkeys consumed soy protein isolates either with or without isoflavones. The researchers found little or no difference between the two groups of monkeys in blood-estrogen level or in the weight of the uterus; an increase in uterine weight is one sign that may indicate cancer.

Cline and colleagues compared the effects of soy protein containing isoflavones with different hormone combinations and with tamoxifen (a drug used to treat breast cancer) on the inner lining of the vagina of surgically postmenopausal monkeys. They found that estrogen, a form of progesterone (another female hormone), a combination of estrogen and progesterone, and tamoxifen all caused some degree of change in the vaginal lining. The soy protein containing isoflavones, on the other hand, had no effect on the vaginal lining. The authors suggested that this study supported the "possibility that soybean estrogens may be a 'tissue-selective' estrogen with minimal effects on the reproductive tract." This means that the phytoestrogens in soy may provide the benefits of estrogens without causing some of the undesirable effects usually associated with estrogens, including changes in the vaginal lining.

Stomach Cancer

Stomach cancer is the tenth leading cause of cancer death in both men and women in the United States. It is expected to cause the deaths of an estimated 7,900 men and 5,600 women in 1999. Limited *in vitro* research has looked at the potential effect of genistein on stomach cancer. Yanagihara and associates found that genistein inhibited the growth of cell lines for stomach cancer.

RESEARCH ON THE SAFETY OF SOY

Research investigating the effects of soy isoflavones on cancer can take one of two approaches. One way is to use foods containing soy protein with its naturally occurring isoflavones. The level of genistein typically used in soy protein-based study diets doesn't lead to any known toxicity and has been consumed by Asian peoples for centuries. The second approach involves the use of purified isoflavones such as might be sold in pills or capsules, which can then be administered in larger amounts than are present in foods. Of course, these higher doses of isoflavones need to be tested in humans for possible side effects not associated with the consumption of soy protein-based foods.

There has also been some concern about the potential of phytoestrogens to stimulate hormone-based cancers. (This topic is briefly discussed on page 33.) A quote from a review article written by respected research scientists Herman Adlercreutz and Witold Mazur adequately puts the concern into perspective: "There is no evidence in the literature suggesting that phyto-oestrogens, present in such amounts in human food that they could have biological effects, stimulate already existing cancer, and there is also no evidence that such phyto-oestrogens could initiate cancer. The high plasma levels in Japanese subjects having low breast, prostate, and colon cancer risk would also suggest that soy consumption is not associated with any risk." These authors also noted that there have been no reports of soy intake affecting fertility in humans.

The recognized safety of using traditional soy protein-based foods as the source of genistein led to the initiation of clinical trials in 1994 to examine the effect of soy protein isolates on cancers of the breast and prostate. These studies are designed to show any potential of soy with naturally occurring isoflavones to help prevent cancer and to identify any possible risk that might be associated with consuming soy.

CONCLUSION

It is now generally accepted that what you eat can affect your risk of developing some types of cancer. In fact, the American Cancer Society estimates that about one-third of the cancer deaths each year are due to dietary factors. Just as some foods and dietary habits are associated with the development of cancer, others have now been shown to help prevent cancer. There is an increasing amount of research supporting the observation from population studies that people consuming appreciable amounts of soyfoods are at lower risk of certain types of cancer, including tumors of the breast, uterus, and prostate. In addition, some *in vitro* studies have shown that genistein helps stop the growth of certain types of stomach cancer cells. Much of the research on soy and cancer has focused on soy isoflavones, which have been found to have several functions that may potentially reduce cancer risk.

4

OSTEOPOROSIS

O steoporosis literally means "porous bones." It is sometimes called the "silent thief" because it robs bones of strength-giving calcium, leaving them weak and brittle. Osteoporosis represents a threat to the health and quality of life of an estimated 25 million Americans and is a major cause of disability. Although typically thought of as occurring in post-menopausal women, osteoporosis can also affect men.

Even though osteoporosis isn't a direct cause of death, don't make the mistake of considering it a minor problem. It leads to 1.5 million broken or fractured bones each year, mostly occurring in the hip, spine, and wrist. One in three women past the age of fifty will suffer a fracture in the bones of the spine (vertebrae), and these numbers are only expected to rise as the population ages. It is estimated that the financial cost of the broken or fractured bones caused by osteoporosis is about $10 billion each year. The good news is that we can take preventive action against osteoporosis. Let's look at osteoporosis in more detail before considering how soy with naturally occurring isoflavones may be able to influence it.

BONE BASICS AND OSTEOPOROSIS

Bones are living tissues made up of two main components. The first is protein-based connective tissue, which provides the somewhat flexible underlying structure of bone. The second component consists of minerals, primarily calcium, that are deposited in the connective tissue and give bone its characteristic hardness.

Contrary to appearances, bones are in a constant state of change. Specialized cells called osteoclasts are constantly breaking down bone, while other cells called osteoblasts are constantly building it back up. The normal, healthy maintenance of bones is a matter of balance between the amount being broken down and the amount being rebuilt. When more bone is broken down than is rebuilt, it becomes weak and easily broken. This is often described as resulting from a loss of bone mineral density. Maximum bone mineral density—the heaviest bone weight—is usually reached around ages thirty to thirty-five. Both men and women begin to experience a small, gradual loss of bone mass by their mid-thirties.

A number of factors affect bone mineral density, including inheritance, diet, aging, hormones, and lifestyle. For example, an individual may inherit the tendency to have small, light-weight bones. Since weight-bearing exercise helps maintain bone mineral density, the American tendency toward physical inactivity also contributes to weaker bones.

Osteoporosis involves the loss of bone mineral density. Probably the most familiar characteristic of osteoporosis is the stooped posture—*dowager's hump*—that results from the collapse of the vertebrae. There is more than one type of osteoporosis. Type I osteoporosis, which is the most common type, occurs in postmenopausal women. Type II (or senile) osteoporosis occurs in both men and women, typically at age seventy and older. Osteoporosis can also be secondary to another illness, or it can result from certain drugs. There is even a rare type of osteoporosis found in children and young adults. The following discussion deals primarily with Type I osteoporosis.

The Calcium Factor

The amount of calcium consumed in the diet and retained in the body throughout life is critical to bone health. Calcium is the most abundant mineral present in the body. About 1 percent is in blood, while the remaining 99 percent is bound up in bone. If there isn't enough calcium in the diet to maintain the level in the blood, which is critical for a number of essential functions, the body steals calcium from its bones. Table 4.1 shows the recommendations for calcium intake made by the National Institutes of Health (NIH) panel. The NIH recommendations reflect a new interest in identifying optimum levels of certain essential nutrients that may actually help prevent diseases, in this case osteoporosis.

As will become clear, the amount of calcium a person consumes is not the only thing to consider. It is also important to take a look at factors that might increase the amount of calcium excreted from the body.

The Protein-Calcium Link

Research suggests that protein and calcium are linked in ways important to the discussion of osteoporosis. The main functions of protein are to build and repair tissue. Once adulthood is reached, under normal circumstances

Table 4.1. Recommended Calcium Intakes to Help Prevent Osteoporosis

Gender	Age Range	Calcium Intake (milligrams)
Males and females	Birth to 6 months	400
	6 months to 1 year	600
	1–5 years	800
	6–10 years	800–1,200
	11–24 years	200–1,500
Men	25–65 years	1,000
	Over 65 years	1,500
Women	25–50 years	1,000
	Pregnant or nursing	1,200–1,500
	Over 50 years (postmenopausal)	
	On estrogen	1,000
	Not on estrogen	1,500
	Over 65 years	1,500

From the National Institiutes of Health's "NIH Consensus Development Panel on Optimal Calcium Intake: Optimal Calcium Intake," *Journal of the American Medical Association* 272 (1994):1942–1948.

the body only needs enough protein to replace the amount lost in the routine protein turnover in the body. Most American adults consume considerably more protein than they need.

An excess of protein can affect other nutrients in the body. For one thing, a number of studies have shown that a high protein intake increases the amount of calcium lost from the body in urine. Research indicates that when protein intake is high, it takes more calcium to achieve a balance between calcium intake and calcium loss in the body. On the other hand, when protein intake is as low as 50 grams per day, it is possible to have a positive calcium balance—less being lost than is being consumed—on a calcium intake as low as 500 to 600 milligrams daily. The fact that Americans consume so much protein may help explain our higher calcium needs.

However, this isn't the whole protein-calcium story. Apparently not all protein has the same effect on calcium excretion. Soy protein has been found to cause less excretion of calcium from the body than animal protein.

The Hormone Factor

Hormones also play an extremely important role in women's bone health. Throughout a woman's reproductive years, estrogen protects her bones by causing them to absorb calcium from her blood and by slowing the loss of calcium from bone. Women don't suddenly stop producing estrogen at menopause. They typically experience decreasing estrogen levels for several years prior to menopause—a period called *perimenopause.* Accelerated bone loss, however, primarily occurs in the fifteen to twenty years following menopause.

Back when women died at a much younger age, spending a few years without estrogen might not have represented a great risk to health. However, women now live much longer; for many American women, the postmenopausal period will represent one-third of their life span. Many women are actively seeking ways to preserve their bone health during these decades after their bodies have essentially stopped producing estrogen. There is a continuing controversy about the benefits versus the risks of estrogen replacement therapy (ERT) and hormone replacement therapy (HRT), the latter consisting of a combination of estrogen with another hormone, typically a form of progesterone.

It is widely accepted that ERT reduces the risk of heart disease and osteoporosis and may even delay or prevent Alzheimer's disease in women. On the other hand, estrogen by itself has a harmful effect on the endometrium (uterine lining), which is one reason why women may prefer HRT to ERT. Although many women are firmly convinced that ERT has been shown to increase the risk of breast cancer, research has not convincingly established this association.

This "good news-bad news" aspect of estrogen replacement has resulted in a lot of concern and confusion among women. A survey by Salamone and associates of older women's attitudes about estrogen replacement was published in 1996. It showed that of the 7,667 women surveyed, 17.4 percent currently were using oral estrogens, 27.2 percent were past users, and 55.4 percent had never used oral estrogen therapy. In spite of the extensive information about the health benefits of ERT, approximately 30 percent of the women who quit using estrogen and 30 percent of the women who had never used estrogen stated that they felt that they didn't need it. And the main reason women gave for not ever starting estrogen therapy was a fear that it was harmful.

Because of this widespread reluctance to use ERT and HRT, there has been increasing emphasis on investigating other approaches that might offer some of the same benefits as ERT and HRT. Logically, some of this interest has focused on the phytoestrogens that occur naturally in some plant foods, especially the isoflavones in soy.

SOY PROTEIN AND OSTEOPOROSIS

Soy protein with naturally occurring isoflavones may potentially play several roles in the prevention of osteoporosis. First, soy protein causes less calcium to be excreted from the body than meat protein. Second, soy isoflavones apparently help preserve bone mineral density without having negative side effects that may be associated with ERT or HRT. And finally, soy's primary isoflavone—genistein—may inhibit the activity of cells that break down bone.

Effect of the Protein in Soy

A study by Breslau and associates looked at the effect on calcium loss of having subjects consume either animal protein or an equal amount of soy protein. Results showed that the animal-protein diet greatly increased calcium excretion compared with soy protein. The authors of the study commented that a diet containing predominantly meat protein may represent a risk for the development of osteoporosis. This suggests that, compared with animal protein, consuming soy protein may help reduce calcium loss and may protect against the development of osteoporosis.

Epidemiologists often look at the rate of hip fracture as a rough indicator of the prevalence of osteoporosis. Oddly enough, those peoples with higher calcium intakes also have higher hip-fracture rates. In their book titled *The Simple Soybean and Your Health,* authors Mark and Virginia Messina present some interesting statistics showing the hip fracture rate (per 100,000 population) and the approximate intakes of calcium and animal protein in a number of locations around the globe (see Table 4.2).

Table 4.2 shows that the hip fracture rate is much higher in Western countries than in Eastern locations. Of course, it is impossible to draw any conclusions about cause and effect from this type of information. However, it is interesting to note that, contrary to what might seem logical, a low calcium intake does not appear to be associated with an increase in hip fractures.

The previous observations about the protein-calcium (see page 31) link may help to explain an apparent paradox. Although Asians typically consume much less calcium than Americans and people in other Western countries, the predominance of plant protein in the Asian diet may help prevent

Table 4.2. Calcium Intake, Animal-Protein Intake, and Rate of Hip Fracture in Selected Locations

Country	Hip-Fracture Rate (per 100,000 population)	Approximate Calcium Intake (mg/day)	Approximate Animal-Protein Intake (grams/day)
Western Nations			
United States	144.9	973	72.0
United Kingdom	118.2	977	56.6
Norway	190.4	1,087	66.6
Eastern Locations			
Singapore	21.6	389	24.7
Hong Kong	45.6	356	34.6

Adapted from *The Simple Soybean and Your Health* by Mark Messina and Virginia Messina.

the greater calcium loss that is associated with a high intake of animal protein.

Effect of the Isoflavones in Soy

A study by Anderson and associates in rats who were surgically postmenopausal showed that an optimal dose of genistein resulted in retaining about the same percent of bone mineral density as when estrogen was administered. Another animal study by Fanti and colleagues indicated that genistein protects rats from the bone loss associated with low estrogen levels, but that its mechanism of action is different than that of estrogen.

Potter and associates conducted a study in postmenopausal women. They compared the effect of consuming soy protein at two levels of naturally occurring isoflavones with consuming the same amount of animal protein (casein). The two soy-protein diets were fortified with calcium to equal the amount provided in the casein diet. This fairly short-term study showed that, compared with the casein group, the women consuming the soy protein diet with the higher level of naturally occurring isoflavones had increases in both bone mineral content and bone mineral density in the lumbar area of the spine.

Effect of Genistein as a Tyrosine Kinase Inhibitor

Osteoclasts, which break down bone, are unusually dependent on the activity of the enzyme tyrosine kinase. This fact led researchers to investigate the effect of genistein—soy's primary isoflavone and a tyrosine kinase inhibitor—on these cells. Both *in vitro* and *in vivo* studies showed that genistein appears to suppress osteoclast function, resulting in a slower breakdown of bone.

CONCLUSION

Osteoporosis is a terribly crippling disease that can greatly decrease a person's quality of life. Fortunately, we can take preventive measures to help preserve our precious bones. Of course, it is essential that you have an adequate calcium intake throughout your lifetime. Then, eating foods that give you the high-quality protein in soy in place of some animal protein may benefit you in several ways. First, the soy protein will allow your body to retain more of the calcium you consume. Next, soy protein with naturally occurring isoflavones may help you preserve the calcium in your bones. Finally, genistein may suppress the activity of the cells that break down bone. When you consider all of the potential health benefits of consuming soy protein with naturally occurring isoflavones—with no known downside—it's hard to understand why everyone hasn't jumped on the soy bandwagon.

5

MENOPAUSE AND MENOPAUSAL SYMPTOMS

Unlike heart disease, cancer, and osteoporosis, which have been discussed in the preceding chapters, menopause is a normal occurrence in the life of every woman who lives long enough. However, the symptoms that women may experience as they decrease estrogen production before and at the time of menopause are much more common in Western women than in Asian women. When researchers sought possible explanations for these differences, they began to focus on the potential effect of the phytoestrogens that occur naturally in soy, which is a staple of most Asian diets.

MENOPAUSE BASICS

Put simply, menopause is a normal stage in a woman's life at which she stops menstruating. It typically occurs between the ages of forty and fifty-five, and the average age at menopause is fifty-one. Although women sometimes think of menopause as an abrupt change, it is normally preceded by perimenopause—a period extending over several years during which there is a gradual decrease in the amount of estrogen produced by the ovaries.

As was discussed in previous chapters, estrogen has a number of benefits that can be lost when levels drop too low. For much of their adult lives, women have a lower risk of heart disease than men the same age. However, once a woman reaches menopause and her estrogen levels fall, her prevalence of cardiovascular disease (CVD) rises to equal and finally surpass that of men. In addition, the risk of osteoporosis in women rises as estrogen levels decrease, both during perimenopause and following menopause. Without estrogen's protective effects, the rate of bone loss is increased; it is highest during the first five to seven years after menopause.

Some women experience few, if any, symptoms at menopause. However, the majority of Western women experience some noticeable symptoms as their estrogen levels decrease. Physical symptoms can include hot flashes, night sweats, and insomnia; changes in vaginal tissues; a decrease in the ability to control urination; headaches; aching and painful joints; and sore breasts. Psychological effects associated with menopause include sudden mood changes; irritability; problems with concentration and memory; anxiety; a feeling of being unable to cope; and even depression.

Hot flashes are sudden feelings of intense heat, which usually last from thirty seconds to five minutes. They often start in the neck and spread upward to the face and scalp, and down to the upper chest. A woman having a hot flash may have a flushed face and sweat profusely. Some women even experience a strong and/or rapid heartbeat and feel dizzy during a hot flash. Hot flashes that occur at night are called night sweats. It is not unusual for a menopausal woman to wake several times during the night with her night clothes and the bed sheets soaking wet. These disturbances contribute greatly to the insomnia that may become a problem at menopause.

Without estrogen, the tissues lining the vagina become thinner and more fragile, and there is a lessening of lubrication. The most common result of this change is discomfort and pain during intercourse. The tissue lining the urinary tract undergoes similar changes, leading to a decrease in the muscle tone that controls the release of urine from the bladder. This inability to control loss is called urinary incontinence.

For some women, menopause is a time of emotional upheaval. Declining estrogen levels may have a direct effect on mood and other feelings. And, of course, insomnia and lack of restful sleep can be major contributors to moodiness, irritability, and the other psychological side effects sometimes associated with menopause.

A survey of 8,000 women conducted in Scotland indicated that 57 percent of the women responding had experienced one or more of the menopausal symptoms mentioned above. This percent is actually lower than the estimates of 70 to 85 percent usually given for North American women. The interesting fact is that Asian women have a much lower incidence of menopausal symptoms. For example, studies estimated that less than 25 percent of Japanese women and 18 percent of Chinese women complained of hot flashes. These observations led researchers to investigate the possible effects on menopausal symptoms of dietary factors in Asian cuisines, including soyfood consumption.

THE POTENTIAL ROLE FOR SOY PROTEIN WITH NATURALLY OCCURRING ISOFLAVONES AS HORMONE REPLACEMENT

There are a growing number of studies investigating the potential effects of soy and soy protein with naturally occurring isoflavones on symptoms and other changes that are associated with menopause. This is an area of intense interest for researchers seeking new treatment options for menopausal women.

The majority of postmenopausal women, who are *not* on ERT or HRT, give a number of reasons for their choice. Some women choose not to start therapy or to discontinue it, either because they don't want to deal with the side effects of HRT, such as continuing menstrual periods, or because they are afraid that it will increase their risk of breast cancer. Other women are advised not to use ERT/HRT by their physicians, usually for the same reasons. This has led to an increasing interest in investigating the possible role of soy protein with naturally occurring isoflavones as a partial or complete replacement for ERT/HRT.

Recent research in monkeys conducted by Clarkson and colleagues has shown that soy protein with naturally occurring isoflavones mimics many of estrogen's activities, but without the negative effects that may accompany ERT or HRT. As the evidence on the positive effects of soy protein containing isoflavones continues to mount, it is possible that these naturally occurring phytoestrogens may be able to play an important role in an alternative form of postmenopausal estrogen replacement.

Effects on Hot Flashes

Of the physical symptoms commonly associated with menopause, hot flashes are perhaps the easiest to measure. In one study by Murkies and associates, postmenopausal women who were regularly experiencing hot flashes were given either soy flour or wheat flour over a three-month period. Although both groups had a decrease in the number of hot flashes they experienced and in their menopausal symptom score, the soy produced a more rapid response.

A recent study by Albertazzi and colleagues in which soy protein with naturally occurring isoflavones was compared with a placebo (casein) in postmenopausal women showed a stronger result. In this study, the researchers found that soy protein was significantly superior to the placebo in reducing the mean number of hot flashes experienced daily. The women taking soy protein had a 26 percent reduction in the mean number of hot flashes by the third week, increasing to a 33 percent reduction by the fourth week, and a 45 percent reduction by the end of the twelfth week.

Effects on Cancer Risk

As was mentioned previously, fear of cancer is a basic reason many women give for not taking ERT or HRT at menopause. Some studies suggest that soy protein with naturally occurring isoflavones preserves bone mineral density and reduces postmenopausal symptoms—two important reasons for taking ERT or HRT—without increasing cancer risk. Furthermore, animal studies have shown that soy isoflavones don't raise hormone concentrations in the blood and don't increase the weight of the uterus, prostate, or testicles. (As discussed in previous chapters, increased weight of an organ is a possible indicator of tumor growth.)

Effects on Cardiovascular Disease

Among the potential benefits that soy has as a hormone replacement is the prevention of CVD. As discussed in Chapter 2, soy protein containing isoflavones reduces blood levels of harmful lipoproteins, acts as an antioxidant, inhibits rapid reproduction of smooth muscle cells, and has other activities that favor a lower risk of atherosclerosis and CVD. ERT has a tendency to increase blood levels of triglyceride, a lipoprotein associated with increased risk of heart disease, especially in women. Soy protein containing isoflavones, however, doesn't increase triglyceride levels.

Also, you may remember that the neurotransmitter acetylcholine causes normal arteries to dilate and atherosclerotic arteries (clogged with plaque) to constrict. ERT enhances the ability of atherosclerotic arteries to dilate in response to acetylcholine. However, the addition of progesterone in HRT somewhat reduces this positive effect. Studies in animals show that soy protein containing isoflavones is comparable to estrogen alone in its ability to dilate atherosclerotic arteries and allow a better blood flow.

CONCLUSION

Menopause is a time of tremendous physical and psychological changes for women. ERT and HRT have helped protect women against some of the negative changes that can occur during menopause. However, the side effects sometimes associated with ERT and HRT and the fear that these therapies may increase cancer risk have caused the majority of women to avoid or discontinue taking them. Research has shown that Asian women who consume large amounts of plant estrogens, especially the isoflavones in soy, have fewer menopausal symptoms and less postmenopausal osteoporosis and CVD than women in the West. This has led to increased interest in evaluating soy with its naturally occurring isoflavones as a possible alternative for ERT or HRT. Although there are many questions still to be answered about the benefits of consuming soy and its phytoestrogens for menopausal women, there would appear to be nothing to lose and potentially a lot to gain by women adding soy to their diets.

6

INCORPORATING SOY (PROTEIN) INTO YOUR DIET

Soy protein is appropriate for just about everyone, with the exception of individuals who are allergic to soy. Millions of Asian peoples have safely consumed soy for thousands of years, and these populations have generally demonstrated a lower risk of many of the chronic diseases that plague the West. The health benefits of soy are becoming more familiar to the American consumer. As a result, soyfoods can now be found in more than half of regular supermarkets. This final chapter provides you with information on available soy products and some tips on making these foods a part of your daily diet.

SOYFOOD OPTIONS

The versatile soybean is the basis for a wide variety of foods. These range from traditional soyfoods to a growing number of new soy protein-based foods. It may be useful to categorize soyfoods into generations.

First Generation Soyfoods

First generation soyfoods are the traditional soyfoods often found in Asian cuisines. Some are mainstream, like tofu and soymilk, while others are often found only in Asian food markets.

Dried Soybeans.   These legumes are most commonly yellow, but can also be brown or black. Black soybeans have a sweet, nutty taste and are considered to be especially delicious. All these types of soybeans can be cooked and used in sauces, casseroles, stews, and soups. Dried soybeans should be available in many supermarkets. Like all dried beans, they must be soaked before cooking.

Green Soybeans, or Edamamé.   Green soybeans are large and sweet. They are harvested when they are still green, then removed from the pod and cooked. They can be served at a meal as a vegetable or eaten as a snack. You may need to go to a specialty food store for green soybeans.

Soymilk. Soymilk serves as a nondairy milk substitute. It is the liquid that remains after soybeans have been soaked, cooked, ground, and strained. You can drink soymilk as a beverage or pour it over cereal. You can also use soymilk as a replacement for cow's milk in the preparation of all types of foods—pancakes, waffles, cream soups and sauces, custards and puddings, and shakes, to name a few.

In addition to finding soymilk in health food and specialty food stores, it may now be available in the dairy case of some supermarkets. Not all soymilks are alike, so check the label for the amount of soy protein and fat in your product. Regular soymilk contains the soybean oil found naturally in soybeans. However, some consumers prefer to purchase the low-fat soymilks that are available. Some brands of soymilk are fortified with calcium, vitamin D, and/or vitamin B_{12}.

Tofu. This soft, cheese-like food is actually soybean curd. Just as cheese is made by curdling milk, tofu is made by coagulating fresh, hot soymilk. It has got to be one of the most versatile forms of soy. In fact, tofu sometimes is called "meat without the bone" because it can be used in place of meat in a variety of dishes. Its growing popularity has also led to tofu being called the "yogurt of the '90s."

There are three main types of tofu—firm, soft, and silken. Firm tofu is preferred for dishes in which you want the tofu to hold its shape—stir-fry dishes, casseroles, soups, or on the grill. Soft tofu and silken tofu are often used in pureed or blended dishes. Tofu has a very bland taste and can absorb the flavors of any foods with which it is mixed. You should be able to find tofu in most supermarkets, in addition to health food and specialty food stores.

Tempeh. A traditional food in Indonesia, tempeh is made from whole soybeans that are sometimes mixed with rice or millet before they are fermented to form a chunky, tender cake. Tempeh has a definite flavor, usually nutty or smoky. It can be used in many of the same ways as firm tofu—marinated and grilled, or as an addition to casseroles, stews, and soups.

Okara. Okara is the solid material—pulp—strained out during the production of soymilk. This soyfood is very high in fiber, but contains very little protein. Since okara has a taste somewhat like coconut, it can be baked or added as a source of fiber to cookies, muffins, or granola. Okara can also be used to make commercial meatless "burger" products.

Miso. If you eat traditional Asian cooking, you have almost certainly been introduced to miso. This rich, salty condiment is made by fermenting a combination of soybeans and either rice or barley to form a paste. Traditionally, miso is aged for several years. Although new chemical processes can produce miso within days, the flavor may not be equal to the aged variety. Miso soup is a popular item in Japanese cuisine, and miso is also used in a variety of their sauces, dressings, and marinades.

Natto. This soy product is made by fermenting cooked, whole soybeans. Its texture is much like cheese, and it has a thick, sticky coating. In Asian countries, natto is traditionally served over rice or as an addition to miso soups or vegetables.

Yuba. Have you ever heated milk to too high a temperature, only to find a "skin" forming over the top of the milk as it cools? The same thing happens when hot soymilk is cooled, and the thin skin is called yuba. Since nothing to do with the soybean is wasted, fresh, half-dried, and dried yuba are available in many Asian food stores. Dried yuba can be deep-fried and eaten as a snack, or it can be added to soups or stews. Soaked in water, softened dried yuba can be used to wrap vegetables or rice.

Soybean Sprouts. Soy sprouts, or soybean sprouts, are traditionally parboiled and added to salads or soups. They are also included in stir-fried, sautéed, or baked dishes.

Second and Third Generation Soyfoods

The second and third generation soyfoods contain soy-based ingredients. Soy flour characterizes the second generation, while textured soy protein represents the third generation of soy products.

Soy Flour. Soy flour is made by roasting soybeans and then grinding them into a fine powder. Natural or full-fat soy flour retains the soybean oil naturally present in soybeans. As the name suggests, defatted soy flour has had the soybean oil removed during processing. Some soy flours are lecithinated, meaning that lecithin has been added. (Lecithin is a fatty compound containing phosphorus, normally manufactured by the body.) Lecithin is added during the manufacture of many different foods because it can act as an emulsifier, allowing fats and oils to be mixed with water-based ingredients, as well as a stabilizer and an antioxidant. It also helps control crystallization and spattering of foods.

Soy flour is high in protein, so adding it to baked goods or to other recipes increases their protein content. Try replacing up to one-fourth of the flour in your baked products with soy flour—an excellent way to increase nutritional content. If you are planning to use only soy flour in your recipe, note that it does not contain gluten—the tough, elastic protein that helps retain the gas bubbles formed by leavening agents, allowing baked goods to rise. Therefore, soy flour should either be combined with wheat flour or have gluten added to it in order to produce a light yeast-raised baked product.

Textured Soy Protein. Textured soy protein (TSP), which has been available for several decades, is an ingredient made from defatted soy flour. The special methods used to cook the soy flour produce a high-protein product that can assume many different forms. When water is added to TSP, for example, it takes on a chewy texture, which makes it ideal for extending or replacing meats. TSP is typically used as the basic ingredient in many products sold as meat substitutes. The term TSP is often used to describe products made from textured soy flour, TSP concentrates, or spun soy fiber.

Some products made from textured soy protein may have lost some or most of their isoflavones in processing. Check to see if the label on a product containing TSP indicates that it has retained the naturally occurring isoflavones.

Table 6.1, adapted from a table developed by Dr. James Anderson, gives the estimated isoflavone content for some first, second, and third generation soy products. It is important to note that the listed values are estimated. Isoflavone content varies widely among varieties of soybeans and from product to product.

Table 6.1. Estimates of Isoflavone Content of Selected Soyfoods

Soyfood	Serving Size	Isoflavone Content (milligrams/serving)
Mature soybeans, uncooked	$\frac{1}{2}$ cup	175.6
Roasted soybeans	$\frac{1}{2}$ cup	167.0
Textured soy protein, dry	$\frac{1}{4}$ cup	93.6
Green soybeans, uncooked	$\frac{1}{2}$ cup	70.1
Tempeh, uncooked	4 ounces	60.5
Soy flour	$\frac{1}{4}$ cup	43.8
Tofu, uncooked	4 ounces	38.3
Soymilk	1 cup	20.0

Adapted with permission from James Anderson, MD. Isoflavone Chart.
www.hcf-nutrition.org/isoflavone_chart.html

Fourth Generation Soyfoods

Some individuals who would like to include soy in their diets have a difficult time consuming adequate amounts of the foods previously discussed. In recent years, however, food manufacturers have developed a growing number of soy-based foods that are more suited to the Western palate. Some are formulated to replace foods already present in the American diet. Others provide quick and easy ways to incorporate soy protein into a daily meal plan. Typically, these fourth generation soyfoods are made with either soy protein concentrates or soy protein isolates.

Food Replacements.   There are quite a few soy products available that can be used to replace familiar non-soy foods. Many of the soy-based products designed to replace dairy foods were originally developed as an option for people who needed to avoid the lactose ("milk sugar") naturally occurring in most dairy products. For example, you can purchase soy-based yogurt, which is made from soymilk. It has a creamy texture that also makes it a good substitute for sour cream and for cream cheese. There are also a number of variations on ice cream, usually providing differing amounts of fat. Soy frozen desserts are typically made from soymilk or soy yogurt. And, of course, a variety of soy-based cheeses are available.

You may also want to try soynut butter. This "other" nut butter is made from crushed, roasted whole soynuts that are blended with soybean oil and other ingredients. Snackers will enjoy trying soynuts (roasted whole soybeans), a high-protein snack containing soy isoflavones.

Fast-and-Easy Soy Food.   "Fast…faster…fastest" seems to have become the motto of much of the West. This "hurry-up" philosophy extends from travel, to communications, and all the way to food. We eat a lot of specialty food products that can be consumed on the run. Not to be outdone, manufacturers of soyfoods have developed a number of convenient-to-eat products that you are sure to enjoy.

Typically, these foods are based on one of the two types of soy-protein food ingredients mentioned in Chapter 1—soy protein concentrates or soy protein isolates (or isolated soy protein). Soy protein isolates, for example, are currently being incorporated into a growing number of products.

Soy beverages aren't the same as soymilk. They can be formulated to provide up to 25 grams of protein per cup and any combination of vitamins and minerals. Various flavors of these soy beverages come in ready-to-drink form or as powdered mixes. You might even want to keep some plain, unsweetened soy-protein powder on hand. It can be added to foods, such as fruit smoothies, or used to add soy-protein power to your cooking. There are also a variety of flavored bars available, allowing you to get your soy protein while you are on the move. You may enjoy munching on some soy-based yogurt-style snacks. And, there are more products currently under development.

In addition to being more familiar to American palates, these new products offer another advantage over some of the more traditional soy-foods. As was mentioned previously, there are several factors that influence the amount of isoflavones in soybeans and the soyfoods made from them. Soy-based foods made from a standardized ingredient, such as soy protein isolates, provide a known and consistent amount of soy isoflavones. Dr. James Anderson, lead author of the meta-analysis of soy protein's effect on cholesterol-lowering (see page 14), commented that those soy products with a standardized amount of genistein "should be selected by women who are seeking the protective effects of soy isoflavones against breast cancer, osteoporosis, or menopausal symptoms." He approximated that consuming 23 to 28 grams of soy protein per day might decrease blood-cholesterol levels by about 7 to 10 percent and reduce estimated risk for coronary heart disease by 15 to 25 percent.

How do you know what type of soy protein ingredient you are getting? Can you tell if it has retained its naturally occurring isoflavones? Probably the best way is to choose products containing a reliable standardized source of soy protein isolates. For example, *Supro* brand soy protein isolates are manufactured by the largest producer of soy protein isolates in the world. The processing methods used in the manufacture of *Supro* leave the naturally occurring isoflavones intact. *Supro* is used as the source of soy protein in the majority of recent research studies, resulting in it having been studied more extensively than any other source of soy protein. Many products containing *Supro* identify this brand of soy protein isolates on their label.

ADDING UP SOY PROTEIN IN YOUR DIET

There are any number of ways you can combine soyfoods to get the minimum 23 to 28 grams of protein recommended by Dr. Anderson. Table 1.1 on page 5 provides the estimated protein content of some basic soyfoods. And, checking the Nutrition Facts portion of the labels on the soyfoods you buy will help you calculate your soy protein intake.

Here are some ideas to get you started on a soy-full week. On day one, you might have $1/2$ cup of firm tofu in a stir-fry, providing about 10 grams of soy protein in just this one dish. Add a cup of soymilk (6.7 grams of protein) and $^1/_2$ cup of green soybeans (11.1 grams of protein) and you have almost 28 grams of soy protein. The next day, add a scoop of soy-protein powder (14 grams or more of protein) to a mixture of puréed fresh fruit to make a delicious fruit smoothie, and snack on $^1/_4$ cup of dry-roasted soynuts (17.0 grams of protein) for at least 31 grams of soy protein. On the third day, you are really on the run and need the "eat-on-the-go" type of soy-foods. You might grab a soy-protein bar (14 grams of protein) and add a scoop of chocolate-flavored soy-protein shake powder to a glass of nonfat milk (14 or more grams of protein in the mix) to get at least 28 grams of soy protein the easy way.

CONCLUSION

It is certainly easier to incorporate soyfoods into your diet today than it was a few years ago. Traditional soyfoods, such as tofu and soymilk, are becoming more recognized and many of these products can now be found in mainstream supermarkets. Those people who want the benefits of soy without learning to bake with soy flour or to prepare tofu can choose from a growing number of soy-based foods, such as flavored soy bars and soy-beverage mixes, that are more familiar to the American palate and lifestyle.

CONCLUSION

It is now widely recommended that people in Western nations, including the United States, routinely substitute plant protein for at least some of the animal protein in their diets. Since soy protein is the only plant protein equal in quality to animal protein, consuming protein-containing soyfoods seems to be a logical choice.

In making dietary decisions, keep the following facts in mind:

- Both men and women—everyone—should be interested in reducing the risk of cardiovascular disease. Consumption of soy protein containing naturally occurring isoflavones offers a safe, healthy way to reduce blood-cholesterol levels, especially in people with higher blood cholesterol.

- Research suggests that consumption of soy protein may have a positive effect on the risk of cancer, especially breast cancer in women and prostate cancer in men.

- Women have additional reasons to consume soy protein containing naturally occurring isoflavones. Preliminary research indicates a possible role of soy protein containing isoflavones in helping to maintain bone mineral density at menopause, thereby reducing the risk of osteoporosis.

- Epidemiologic data and some early study results also suggest that soy protein isoflavones may help reduce menopausal symptoms.

And adding soy protein to your diet is easier today than ever before. You should have no problem finding several taste-tempting soy-based foods, including both traditional soyfoods and the bars, beverages, snacks, and other handy new food products that contain soy protein isolates with intact isoflavones.

GLOSSARY

Acetylcholine. A neurotransmitter, which, among other functions, causes normal arteries to dilate (enlarge), and, in most cases, atherosclerotic arteries to constrict.

Angiogenesis. The development of tiny blood vessels to nourish new growth.

Antioxidant. A substance that reduces or prevents oxidation. *See also* Oxidation.

Atherosclerosis. A process in which deposits of cholesterol and other substances build up on and inside an artery wall, making it thick and irregular. Narrowed portions of the artery are more likely to become blocked, cutting off the flow of blood that supplies oxygen and nutrients to cells and tissues.

Benign prostatic hypertrophy (or hyperplasia), or BPH. A noncancerous (benign) enlargement of the prostate gland.

Cancer. A large group of diseases all characterized by cells that grow and multiply in an uncontrolled manner.

Carcinogen. The general term for anything that can produce cancer.

Cardiovascular disease (CVD). A general term for diseases of the heart and blood vessels. CVD includes heart attack, stroke, high blood pressure, and rheumatic heart disease.

Casein. The primary protein in dairy foods.

Cholesterol. A fat-like substance that is necessary in the human body; however, high levels in the blood increase the risk of heart disease. In addition to being produced by the body, cholesterol can also be obtained from eating animal foods.

Daidzein. A phytoestrogen; the second most plentiful isoflavone in soy.

Epidemiology. The study of the causes, distribution, and control of disease in populations.

Estradiol. A very potent form of the hormone estrogen.

Estrogen replacement therapy (ERT). Consists of taking estrogen to replace that lost at natural or surgical menopause.

Fiber. A type of complex carbohydrate that is not digested or absorbed by the human body.

Genistein. A phytoestrogen; the primary isoflavone in soy.

Globulin. A specific type of protein.

Heart attack. Occurs when an artery in the heart is blocked, allowing the cells in the part of the heart supplied with oxygen and nutrients by that artery to be damaged and even die. Heart attack is most often caused by the blockage of an artery already narrowed by atherosclerosis. It can also result from an artery that is blocked when it contracts—goes into spasm.

High-density lipoprotein (HDL). A small particle made up of fat and protein. HDL differs from low-density lipoprotein in that it is not a risk factor for cardiovascular disease. In fact, a high level of HDL actually helps reverse your risk for cardiovascular disease.

Hormone replacement therapy (HRT). Term commonly used to describe therapy consisting of estrogen replacement therapy plus another hormone, typically progesterone or its synthetic form, progestin.

Hormones. Chemical substances produced in one part of the body and carried in the blood to another part of the body where they alter body function.

Isoflavone. A type of phytochemical. Soybeans are the primary source of isoflavones in the human diet.

Lipoprotein. A particle made up of fat ("lipid") and protein. *See also* High-density lipoprotein; Low-density lipoprotein.

Low-density lipoprotein (LDL). A particle made up of fat, mostly cholesterol, and protein. A high level of LDL is a risk factor for cardiovascular disease.

Menopause. The point in a woman's life when she stops menstruating.

Meta-analysis. A research technique that uses statistical methods to combine the results of several different studies. It is often used to combine the results of similar small studies, which, when taken alone, might not be considered large enough to be of significance.

Metastasis. The process by which a disease is spread from its original site to other locations in the body. The term is often used to describe the spread of cancer.

Miso. A rich, salty condiment made by fermenting soybeans and grain; used to flavor a variety of foods in Asian cuisines.

Natto. A cheese-like food made by fermenting cooked, whole soybeans.

Neurotransmitters. Chemical agents produced by "excited" nerve cells in the body. They transmit nerve impulses by crossing the tiny space (synapse) between nerve cells and stimulating the next cell in the nerve.

Okara. A high-fiber by-product of soymilk production.

Osteoblasts. Specialized cells in bone that are constantly breaking it down.

Osteoclasts. Specialized cells in bone that are constantly building it back up.

Osteoporosis. A disease in which bones become extremely weak and are more likely to break as a result of decreased bone mineral density. In many cases, osteoporosis results from the reduction in estrogen that occurs at menopause.

Oxidation. A chemical reaction in which oxygen reacts with another substance. Oxidation can damage particles (such as low-density lipoproteins), cells, and tissues in the body.

Perimenopause. The three to five year period prior to menopause during which estrogen levels begin to drop.

Phytochemical. "Plant chemical"; a term used for thousands of compounds found in plant foods.

Phytoestrogens. Compounds with some estrogen-like activities that are found in plant foods.

Restenosis. The reappearance of narrowing in an artery after angioplasty or other repairs.

Soy flour. An ingredient made by grinding roasted soybeans into a fine powder; it is about 50 percent protein.

Soy protein concentrate. A soy-protein ingredient made from defatted soy flakes; it is about 65 to 70 percent protein.

Soy protein isolate (isolated soy protein). The most highly refined soy-protein ingredient; it is at least 90 percent protein.

Soymilk. A beverage made by soaking, grinding, and straining cooked soybeans.

Stroke. Occurs when an artery supplying blood to the brain is blocked. The damage resulting from an insufficient supply of blood may include a loss of mental function, muscle function, vision, sensation, or speech, depending on the area of the brain that is affected.

Tempeh. Tender fermented soybean cakes.

Textured soy protein (TSP). An ingredient made from defatted soy flour. The term is often used to describe products made from textured soy flour, textured soy protein concentrates, or spun soy fiber.

Tofu. Soybean curd; a soft food that is somewhat similar to cheese in consistency and is made by curdling fresh, hot soymilk with a coagulant.

Trypsin. An enzyme that plays a role in protein digestion.

Yuba. The dried product made from the "skin" that forms on the surface of heated soymilk as it cools.

REFERENCES

Adlercreutz CHT, Goldin BR, Gorbach SL, et al. "Soybean phytoestrogen intake and cancer risk." *Journal of Nutrition* 125 (Suppl 3) (1995): 757S–770S.

Adlercreutz H. "Phytoestrogens: epidemiology and a possible role in cancer protection." *Environmental Health Perspectives* 103 (Suppl 7) (1995): 103–112.

Adlercreutz H, Mazur W. "Phyto-oestrogens and Western diseases." *Annals of Medicine* 29 (1997): 95–120.

Albertazzi P, Pansini F, Bonaccorsi G, et al. "The effect of dietary soy supplementation on hot flushes." *Obstetrics and Gynecology* 91 (1998): 6–11.

American Cancer Society. *Cancer Facts & Figures—1998.* Publication 98-300M-No. 5008.98. Atlanta: American Cancer Society, 1998.

American Cancer Society. *Cancer Facts & Figures—1999.* www.cancer.org/statistics/cff99.

American Heart Association. *1999 Heart and Stroke Statistical Update,* Publication 55-0529, 11-98, 96 08 08 C. Dallas: American Heart Association, 1998.

American Heart Association. *Heart and Stroke Facts,* Publication 55-0523, 11-96, 96 08 08 B. Dallas: American Heart Association, 1996.

Anderson JJB, Garner SC, Ambrose WW, Ohue T. "Genistein and bone: studies in rat models and bone cell lines [meeting abstract]," presented at Second International Symposium on the Role of Soy in Preventing and Treating Chronic Disease, Brussels, Belgium. September 15–18, 1996.

Anderson JW. "Health benefits of soy." *Abstracts of Health Benefits of Soy Protein, 1996,* http://www.ag.uiuc.edu/~stratsoy/soyhealth.html, (accessed July 5, 1998).

Anderson JW, Johnstone BM, Cook-Newell ME. "Meta-analysis of the effects of soy protein intake on serum lipids." *New England Journal of Medicine* 333 (1995): 276–282.

Anthony MS, Clarkson TB, Bullock BC, Wagner JD. "Soy protein versus soy phyto-estrogens in the prevention of diet-induced coronary artery atherosclerosis of male cynomolgus monkeys." *Arteriosclerosis, Thrombosis and Vascular Biology* 17 (1997): 2524–2531.

Anthony MS, Clarkson TB, Hughes CL Jr., et al. "Soybean isoflavones improve cardiovascular risk factors without affecting the reproductive system of peripubertal rhesus monkeys." *Journal of Nutrition* 126 (1996): 43–50.

Bakhit RM, Klein BP, Essex-Sorlie D, et al. "Intake of 25 g of soybean protein with or without soybean fiber alters plasma lipids in men with elevated cholesterol concentrations." *Journal of Nutrition* 124 (1994): 213–222.

Barnes S. "Evolution of the health benefits of soy isoflavones." *Proceedings of the Society for Experimental Biology and Medicine* 217 (1998): 386–392.

Barnes S, Peterson TG, Coward L. "Rationale for the use of genistein-containing soy matrices in chemoprevention trials for breast and prostate cancer." *Journal of Cellular Biochemistry* 22 (Suppl) (1995): 181–187.

Barrett J. "Phytoestrogens. Friends or foes?" *Environmental Health Perspectives* 104 (1996): 478–482.

Berkow R, Beers MH, Fletcher AJ (eds). *The Merck Manual of Medical Information.* Whitehouse Station, New Jersey: Merck Research Laboratories, 1997.

Blair HC. "Action of genistein and other tyrosine kinase inhibitors in preventing osteoporosis [meeting abstract]," presented at Second International Symposium on the Role of Soy in Preventing and Treating Chronic Disease, Brussels, Belgium. September 15–18, 1996.

Breslau NA, Brinkley L, Hill KD, Pak CYC. "Relationship of animal protein-rich diet to kidney stone formation and calcium metabolism." *Journal of Clinical Endocrinology and Metabolism* 66 (1988): 140–146.

Clarkson TB, Anthony MS, Williams JK, et al. "The potential of soybean phytoestrogens for postmenopausal hormone replacement therapy." *Proceedings of the Society for Experimental Biology and Medicine* 217 (1998): 365–368.

Cline JM, Paschold JC, Anthony MS, et al. "Effects of hormonal therapies and dietary soy phytoestrogens on vaginal cytology in surgically postmenopausal macaques." *Fertility and Sterility* 65 (1996): 1031–1035.

Crouse JR III, Terry JG, Morgan TM, et al. "Soy protein containing isoflavones reduces plasma concentrations of lipids and lipoproteins [abstract]." *Circulation* 97 (1998): 816.

Fanti O, Faugere MC, Gang Z, et al. "Systemic administration of genistein partially prevents bone loss in ovariectomized rats in a non-estrogen-like mechanism [meeting abstract]. *American Journal of Clinical Nutrition* 68 (Supplement) (1998): 1517S.

Fotsis T, Pepper MS, Aktas E, et al. "Flavonoids, dietary-derived inhibitors of cell proliferation and *in vitro* angiogenesis." *Cancer Research* 57 (1997): 2916–2921.

Geller J, Sionit L, Partido C, et al. "Genistein inhibits the growth of human-patient BPH and prostate cancer in histoculture." *The Prostate* 34 (1998): 75–79.

Goodman MT, Wilkens LR, Hankin JH, et al. "Association of soy and fiber consumption with the risk of endometrial cancer." *American Journal of Epidemiology* 146 (1997): 294–306.

Gu F-L, Xia T-L, Kong X-T. "Preliminary study of the frequency of benign prostatic hyperplasia and prostatic cancer in China." *Urology* 44 (1994): 688–691.

Guthrie JR, Dennerstein L, Hopper JL, Burger HG. "Hot flushes, menstrual status, and hormone levels in a population-based sample of midlife women." *Obstetrics and Gynecology* 88 (1996): 437–442.

Hawrylewicz EJ, Zapata JJ, Blair WH. "Soy and experimental cancer: animal studies." *Journal of Nutrition* 125 (Suppl 3) (1995): 698S–708S.

Hegsted M, Linkswiler HM. "Long-term effects of level of protein intake on calcium metabolism in young adult women." *Journal of Nutrition* 111 (1981): 244–251.

Hegsted M, Schuette SA, Zemel MB, Linkswiler HM. "Urinary calcium and calcium balance in young men as affected by level of protein and phosphorus intake." *Journal of Nutrition* 111 (1981): 553–562.

Henley EC, Kuster JM. "Protein quality evaluation by protein digestibility-corrected amino acid scoring." *Food Technology* 48 (1994): 74–77.

Honoré EK, Williams JK, Anthony MS. "Enhancement of coronary vasodilation by soy phytoestrogens and genistein [meeting abstract]." *Circulation* 92 (Suppl 1) (1995): I-349.

Honoré EK, Williams JK, Anthony MS, Clarkson TB. "Effects of dietary soy isoflavones on coronary vasodilation, and neointimal formation after iliac artery balloon injury, in atherosclerotic monkeys [meeting abstract]," presented at National Center for Toxicological Research, FDA, 3rd International Conference on Phytoestrogens, Little Rock, Arkansas. December, 1995.

Honoré EK, Williams JK, Anthony MS, Clarkson TB. "Soy isoflavones enhance coronary vascular reactivity in atherosclerotic female macaques." *Fertility and Sterility* 67 (1997): 148–154.

Indiana Soybean Board. *U.S. 1998 Soyfoods Directory.* Lebanon (Indiana): Indiana Soybean Board, 1998.

Kapiotis S, Hermann M, Held I, et al. "Genistein, the dietary-derived angiogenesis inhibitor, prevents LDL oxidation and protects endothelial cells from damage by atherogenic LDL." *Arteriosclerosis, Thrombosis & Vascular Biology* 17 (1997): 2868–2874.

Knight DC, Eden JA. "A review of the clinical effects of phytoestrogens." *Obstetrics & Gynecology* 87 (1996): 897–904.

Lamartiniere CA, Moore JB, Brown NM, et al. "Genistein suppresses mammary cancer in rats." *Carcinogenesis* 16 (1995): 2833–2840.

Lamartiniere CA, Murrill WB, Manzolillo PA, et al. "Genistein alters the ontogeny of mammary gland development and protects against chemically-induced mammary cancer in rats." *Proceedings of the Society for Experimental Biology and Medicine* 217 (1998): 358–364.

Linkswiler HM, Zemel MB, Hegsted M, Schuette S. "Protein-induced hypercalciuria." *Federation Proceedings* 40 (1981): 2429–2433.

Lovati MR, Manzoni C, Corsini A, et al. "Low density lipoprotein receptor activity is modulated by soybean globulins in cell culture." *Journal of Nutrition* 122 (1992): 1971–1978.

Lu L-JW, Anderson KE, Grady JJ, Nagamani M. "Effects of soya consumption for one month on steroid hormones in premenopausal women: implications for breast cancer risk reduction." *Cancer Epidemiology, Biomarkers & Prevention* 5 (1996): 63–70.

Messina M, Messina V, Setchell K. *The Simple Soybean and Your Health.* Garden City Park, New York: Avery Publishing Group, 1994.

Messina MJ, Persky V, Setchell KDR, Barnes S. "Soy intake and cancer risk: a review of the *in vitro* and *in vivo* data." *Nutrition and Cancer* 21 (1994): 113–131.

Murkies AL, Lombard C, Strauss BJG, et al. "Dietary flour supplementation decreases post-menopausal hot flushes: effect of soy and wheat." *Maturitas* 21 (1995): 189–195.

Naik HR, Lehr JE, Pienta KJ. "An *in vitro* and *in vivo* study of antitumor effects of genistein on hormone refractory prostate cancer." *Anticancer Research* 14 (1994): 2617–2620.

National Institutes of Health. "NIH Consensus Development Panel on Optimal Calcium Intake: Optimal calcium intake." *Journal of the American Medical Association* 272 (1994): 1942–1948.

National Report on Consumer Attitudes about Nutrition. Seattle: United Soybean Board, 1997.

Nestel PJ, Yamashita T, Sasahara T, et al. "Soy isoflavones improve systemic arterial compliance but not plasma lipids in menopausal and perimenopausal women." *Arteriosclerosis, Thrombosis and Vascular Biology* 17 (1997): 3392–3398.

NIH Consensus Development Panel on Optimal Calcium Intake. "Optimal calcium intake." *Journal of the American Medical Association* 272 (1994): 1942–1948.

Nilausen K, Meinertz H. "Variable lipemic response to dietary soy protein in healthy, normolipemic men." *American Journal of Clinical Nutrition* 68 (Supplement) (1998): 1380S–1384S.

Peterson G, Barnes S. "Genistein inhibits both estrogen and growth factor-stimulated proliferation of human breast cancer cells." *Cell Growth & Differentiation* 7 (1996): 1345–1351.

Porter M, Penney GC, Russell D, et al. "A population based survey of women's experience of the menopause." *British Journal of Obstetrics and Gynaecology* 103 (1996): 1025–1028.

Potter SM, Baum JA, Teng H, et al. "Soy protein and isoflavones: their effects on blood lipids and bone density in postmenopausal women." *American Journal of Clinical Nutrition* 68 (Supplement) (1998): 1375S–1379S.

Potter SM. "Overview of proposed mechanisms for the hypocholesterolemic effect of soy." *Journal of Nutrition* 125 (Suppl 3) (1995): 606S–611S.

Raines EW, Ross R. "Biology of atherosclerotic plaque formation: possible role of growth factors in lesion development and the potential impact of soy." *Journal of Nutrition* 125 (Suppl 3) (1995): 624S–630S.

Rossi A, DiSilvestro RA, Blostein-Fujii A. "Effects of soy consumption on exercise-induced acute muscle damage and oxidative stress in young adult males [meeting abstract]." *The Federation of American Societies for Experimental Biology Journal* 12 (1998): A653.

Salamone LM, Pressman AR, Seeley DG, Cauley JA. "Estrogen replacement therapy. A survey of older women's attitudes." *Archives of Internal Medicine* 156 (1996): 1293–1297.

Schleicher R, Zheng M, Zhang M, Lamartiniere CA. "Genistein inhibition of prostate cancer cell growth and metastasis in vivo [meeting abstract]." *American Journal of Clinical Nutrition* 68 (Supplement) (1998): 1526S.

Schuette SA, Linkswiler HM. "Effects on Ca and P metabolism in humans by adding meat, meat plus milk, or purified proteins plus Ca and P to a low protein diet." *Journal of Nutrition* 112 (1982): 338–349.

Soybean usage for soyfoods production in the United States (1980–1996). Bar Harbor, Maine: Soyatech, Inc., 1997.

Stoll BA. "Eating to beat breast cancer: potential role for soy supplements." *Annals of Oncology* 8 (1997): 223–225.

Strange CJ. "Boning up on osteoporosis," in *Your Guide to Women's Health,* 3rd edition. DHHS Publication No. (FDA) 97-1181. Rockville (Maryland): Food and Drug Administration, 1997.

Tang GWK. "The climacteric of Chinese factory workers." *Maturitas* 19 (1994): 177–182.

Tierney LM Jr., McPhee SJ, Papadakis MA (eds). *Current Medical Diagnosis & Treatment 1998,* 37th edition. Stamford, Connecticut: Appleton & Lange, 1998.

Tikkanen MJ, Wähälä, K, Ojala S, et al. "Effect of soybean phytoestrogen intake on low density lipoprotein oxidation resistance." *Proceedings of the National Academy of Sciences* 95 (1998): 3106–3110.

Wei H, Wei L, Frenkel K, et al. "Inhibition of tumor promoter-induced hydrogen peroxide formation *in vitro* and *in vivo* by genistein." *Nutrition and Cancer* 20 (1993): 1–12.

Wilcox JN, Blumenthal BF. "Thrombotic mechanisms in atherosclerosis: potential impact of soy proteins." *Journal of Nutrition* 125 (Suppl 3) (1995): 631S–638S.

Yanagihara K, Ito A, Toge T, Numoto M. "Antiproliferative effects of isoflavones on human cancer cell lines established from the gastrointestinal tract." *Cancer Research* 53 (1993): 5815–5821.

Zava DT, Duwe G. "Estrogenic and antiproliferative properties of genistein and other flavonoids in human breast cancer cells *in vitro.*" *Nutrition and Cancer* 27 (1997): 31–40.

Zhang R, Li Y, Wang W. "Enhancement of immune function in mice fed high doses of soy daidzein." *Nutrition and Cancer* 29 (1997): 24–28.

Zhou Y, Lee AS. "Mechanism of the suppression of the mammalian stress response by genistein, an anticancer phytoestrogen from soy." *Journal of the National Cancer Institute* 90 (1998): 381–388.

ABOUT THE AUTHOR

Mary Carole McMann is a registered dietitian, licensed in the state of Texas. After receiving her Bachelor of Science and Master of Public Health degrees, Mary spent much of her career as a research dietitian, nutrition counselor, and health/nutrition writer in her native Oklahoma. She then joined the staff of Baylor College of Medicine in Houston, Texas, where, in addition to working as a research dietitian, she was major contributing author for *The New Living Heart Diet* and four other books in *The Living Heart* series. Since establishing *Marimac Communications* (marimac@flash.net) in Houston in 1996, Mary has written numerous monographs, slide presentations, articles, pamphlets, and brochures for physicians and other health-care professionals, as well as for the public. One of Mary's projects—a monograph on soy protein and coronary heart disease—has been translated into Japanese and into Spanish for Central and South America.

INDEX

Soy protein, 5–7
   antioxidant effects of, 16–17, 22
   effects on artery dilation, 17–18
   effects on atherosclerosis, 17
   effects on blood clotting, 18
   effects on calcium, 31–32
   effects on cancer, 20–29, 39–40
   effects on cardiovascular disease, 40
   effects on cholesterol, 14–17
   effects on immune system function, 22
   effects on menopause, 38–40
   effects on menstrual cycle, 24–25
   effects on osteoporosis, 34–35
   effects on restenosis, 18
   effects on smooth muscle cells, 18
   as hormone replacement therapy, 38–40
   incorporating it into your diet, 41–47
   quality of, 7
   safety of, 28
Soy protein concentrates, 6
Soy protein isolates. *See* Isolated soy protein.
Soybean sprouts, 43
Soybeans
   dried, 41
   green, 41
Soyfoods, 41–47
Soymilk, 42
Soy-protein powder, 45–46
Supro, 46

Tempeh, 42
Textured soy protein (TSP), 44
Tofu, 42
Tyrosine kinases, 24, 35–36

Yuba, 43

POSTSCRIPT

In May 1998, Protein Technologies International submitted a petition to the FDA requesting authorization of a health claim on the association between soy protein and the reduced risk of coronary heart disease. (A health claim is any statement that characterizes the relationship between any nutrient or other substance in a food and a disease or health-related condition.) The petition was supported by data from more than fifty clinical trials. Based on its review of the data, the FDA concluded that there was significant scientific agreement that "consuming 25 grams of soy protein daily, as part of a diet low in saturated fat and cholesterol, may reduce the risk of heart disease." According to the rule proposed by the FDA, food products that contain a minimum of 6.25 grams of soy protein per serving can carry this health claim on their labels. The soy protein health claim was authorized late in October 1999.

The authorization of this health claim is important in several ways. The health claim is a powerful tool to increase public knowledge about the potential health benefits of soy protein. And, it should add considerable impetus to the development of additional soy protein–based foods, making it increasingly easier for individuals to achieve the minimum recommended intake of 25 grams of soy protein per day.